MICH 

M.D.

DISSEMINATED INTRAVASCULAR COAGULATION IN MAN

DISSEMINATED INTRAVASCULAR COAGULATION IN MAN

By

JOHN D. MINNA, M.D.
Chief, Section of Somatic Cell Genetics
Laboratory of Biochemical Genetics
National Heart and Lung Institute
National Institute of Health
Bethesda, Maryland

STANLEY J. ROBBOY, M.D.
Assistant Professor of Pathology
Harvard Medical School
Assistant Pathologist
Massachusetts General Hospital
Boston, Massachusetts

ROBERT W. COLMAN, M.D.
Associate Professor of Medicine and Pathology
University of Pennsylvania Medical School
Chief, Coagulation Unit
Section of Hematology
Hospital of the University of Pennsylvania,
Philadelphia, Pennsylvania

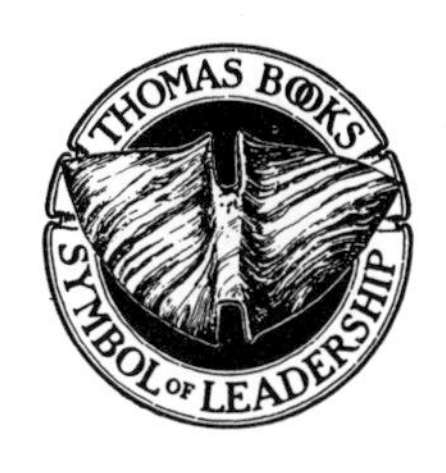

CHARLES C THOMAS • PUBLISHER
Springfield, Illinois, USA

Published and Distributed Throughout the World by
CHARLES C THOMAS • PUBLISHER
Bannerstone House
301-327 East Lawrence Avenue, Springfield, Illinois, U.S.A.

ISBN 0-398-02992-X
Library of Congress Catalog Card Number: 73-14507

With THOMAS BOOKS *careful attention is given to all details of manufacturing and design. It is the Publisher's desire to present books that are satisfactory as to their physical qualities and artistic possibilities and appropriate for their particular use.* THOMAS BOOKS *will be true to those laws of quality that assure a good name and good will.*

Printed in the United States of America

BB-14

Library of Congress Cataloging in Publication Data

Minna, John D
Disseminated intravascular coagulation in man.

Bibliography: p.
1. Disseminated intravascular coagulation.
I. Robboy, Stanley J., joint author. II. Colman, Robert W., joint author. III. Title.
[DNLM: 1. Disseminated intravascular coagulation.
WH310.M665d 1974]
RC647.D5M56 616.1'5 73-14507
ISBN 0-398-02992-X

For

Myrna, Anita, and Roberta

FOREWORD

DISSEMINATED INTRAVASCULAR COAGULATION

Disseminated intravascular coagulation is
a name that stimulates the scientist's imagination. It's
as lovely a disease as ever plagued a human nation,
and charmed a hematologist with fatal fascination.

O thrombin! Mighty enzyme, in excess is seen to circulate
and causes dreadful clots in our anatomy to percolate,
consolidates the platelet plug through viscous metamorphosis
(releasing phospholipid like a bunch of spouting porpoises),
by action on fibrinogen produces fibrin monomer,
which, forming polymer, makes all our situation solemner.
Our physiognomy reacts to this with animosity and well
it might, it's suffering from overdone thrombosity.

Then plasmin. Every bit as powerful, but thrombin's nemesis.
First Enzyme of fibrinolytic mechanism's genesis
reacts with kallikreinogen to change it into kallikrein
and activated bradykinin, results that are vasodilatine.
The aggregate and sticky mass are savagely invaded
so that all that's left of fibrin is disgracefully degraded.
The victim clots like crazy but bleeds like a hemophiliac,
a combination to delight an avid necrophiliac.

And so our lab is researching with selfless dedication,
while digging into people's veins with due precipitation
and administering heparin with dauntless trepidation
and annihilating rabbits without any hesitation.
But one day, either by holy or cerebral divination
we will stumble on, or formulate, the noble preparation
that shall resurrect the ill,
thorough, and efficient, will
put an end to all our sorrow and our tearful tribulation
with disseminated intravascular coagulation.

Sharona BenTov

ACKNOWLEDGMENTS

WE ARE INDEBTED TO THE MEDICAL and pathology house officers of the Massachusetts General Hospital, whose careful observations and high standards of patient care made this study possible. Dr. Alexander Leaf, chairman of the Department of Medicine, Dr. Benjamin Castleman, chairman of the Department of Pathology, and Dr. William Beck, chief of the Clinical Laboratories encouraged and supported us in this endeavor. Drs. Bernard Jacobson, Barbara Rosen, Allan Sandler, and John Truman kindly permitted us to examine their patients. Dr. Sidney Rieder, chief of the Clinical Chemistry Laboratories, and Dr. Lawrence Kunz, chief of the Bacteriology Laboratories, graciously permitted us to review many of their files.

Drs. Norman Birndorf, Jerry Gajewski, Stephen Niewiarowski, Liberto Pechet, and Donald Shapiro read parts of the manuscript and made many helpful suggestions. Miss Paula Giannusa and Miss Lugenia Oxley performed all of the coagulation tests. Mr. Frank McCarthy performed the photography. Miss Arlene Lavallee and Mrs. Helmie Carpenter helped with the manuscript.

During the preparation of this book, we have been partially supported by USPHS Grants HL11519 and HL13206, a junior faculty fellowship from the American Cancer Society to Dr. Robboy, and a career development award (HL48075) to Dr. Colman. Dr. Minna is a member of the U.S. Public Health Service and is grateful to Dr. Marshal Nirenberg for his support. The views presented in this book are not necessarily those of the USPHS or the National Institutes of Health.

PREFACE

ACQUIRED DISORDERS OF BLEEDING and thrombosis are noted with increasing frequency in hospital based medicine. In part, this is related to the growing number of patients with debilitating diseases who survive longer periods because of advances in medical care. Progress in artificial ventilation, use of vasopressors, intense antibiotic therapy, more daring surgical approaches, cancer chemotherapy and successful treatment of cardiovascular and renal disorders have led to increasing numbers of patients with prolonged critical illnesses.

Although many of the acquired hemostatic disorders are related to iatrogenic suppression of platelet production, liver disease and vitamin K deficiency, systemic problems of clot formation and lysis are being recognized with increasing frequency; these generally are categorized under the names disseminated intravascular coagulation (DIC), defibrination syndrome, and consumption coagulopathy.

In the clinical care of acutely ill patients with DIC, recurrent problems of recognition, diagnosis, treatment, prognosis and complications arise.

This monograph represents an attempt to collect prospectively and analyze the clinical data from a large number of patients with DIC cared for by the staff of the Massachusetts General Hospital. The majority of the clinicopathologic observations were made by the authors. The laboratory tests chosen for analysis represent those available generally to the practicing physician.

We have tried to focus on clinical problems and questions of clinicopathologic correlation that the physician faces in dealing with these patients when the only clinical data available is that collected at the bedside. While the final molecular mechanisms involved in hemostasis have yet to be elucidated, there are many practical clinical points that can be made from analyzing our patient data.

Abbreviated clinical histories are used to illustrate these points and bring generalizations based on statistics back to the bedside of the individual patient.

We hope that our conclusions and guideline will aid house officers, internists, surgeons and hematologists who are forced to deal with and make prompt therapeutic decisions in life threatening disorders of hemostasis in the critically ill patient.

John D. Minna
Stanley J. Robboy
Robert W. Colman

ABBREVIATIONS

CNS	central nervous system
CSF	cerebrospinal fluid
CVP	central venous pressure
CT	whole blood clotting time
DIC	disseminated intravascular coagulation
EACA	epsilon aminocaproic acid
ELT	euglobulin clot lysis time
FDP	fibrin(ogen) degradation products
Fi	Fi test for FDP
HCT	hematocrit
HPF	high power field
LDH	lactic dehydrogenase
MGH	Massachusetts General Hospital
MW	molecular weight
PT	prothrombin time
PTT	partial thromboplastin time
RBC	red blood cell
SCT	staphylococcal clumping test for FDP
SGOT	serum glutamic oxalacetic transaminase
SGPT	serum glutamic pyruvic transaminase
TT	thrombin time
TTP	thrombotic (thrombohemolytic) thrombocytopenic purpura
TRCHII	tanned red cell hemagglutination inhibition test for FDP
WBC	white blood cell

CONTENTS

DISSEMINATED INTRAVASCULAR COAGULATION IN MAN

Chapter I

WHAT IS DIC?

HISTORY

DISSEMINATED INTRAVASCULAR COAGULATION (DIC) is a pathological syndrome in which the formation of fibrin thrombi, the consumption of specific plasma proteins, the loss of platelets, and the activation of the fibrinolytic system suggest the presence of thrombin in the systemic circulation. Clinically these effects can become manifest as diffuse hemorrhage and, less frequently, as thrombosis.

For many years clinicians have been aware of an acquired bleeding disorder characterized by severe bleeding and multiple coagulation abnormalities including hypofibrinogenemia (44), but the etiology of the syndrome was usually attributed to excessive fibrinolysis. The concept of DIC was not easily accepted despite data indicating that it was the pathogenic mechanism in abruptio placenta (182), mismatched blood transfusions (98), and that purpura fulminans could be treated successfully with heparin (106).

Extensive studies by Lasch and his associates (101) helped define the syndrome, after which several major works published in 1965–67 spotlighted DIC as an intermediary mechanism of disease (80,115,130,177,208). McKay (115) described much of the pathophysiological foundation characterizing the syndrome, while Hardaway (80) emphasized the importance of acidosis and shock. Rodriguez-Erdman (177) attempted to define the coagulation abnormalities and Verstraete *et al.* (208) emphasized the efficacy of heparin and the protean etiologies. Then Merskey *et al.* (130) introduced the first sensitive method for measuring fibrinogen degradation products (FDP), and the stimulus was provided for clinicians to search for, recognize, and treat DIC.

Since these investigators have reviewed extensively the earlier work on DIC, this chapter will deal with the experience and knowledge accrued since 1965. Emphasis is placed on the pathophysiology of the syndrome and especially upon the biochemical pathways and systems involved. The plan of the prospective clinical pathologic study will also be indicated.

PATHOGENESIS

At least three types of injury may activate the coagulation system (36): (a) injury to the endothelial cell, which by exposing the underlying collagen (215) activates Hageman factor and subsequently the intrinsic clotting system; (b) tissue injury, which by releasing tissue thromboplastin present in the vessel wall (145) in the presence of factor VII, activates the extrinsic clotting system; and (c) red cell, leukocyte or platelet injury, which results in the increased availability of phospholipid, a component needed for the proper functioning of both the intrinsic and extrinsic clotting systems (Fig. I-1). The outcome of these initiating mechanisms is the formation of factor Xa which converts prothrombin to thrombin in the circulating blood and results in the formation of fibrin. It

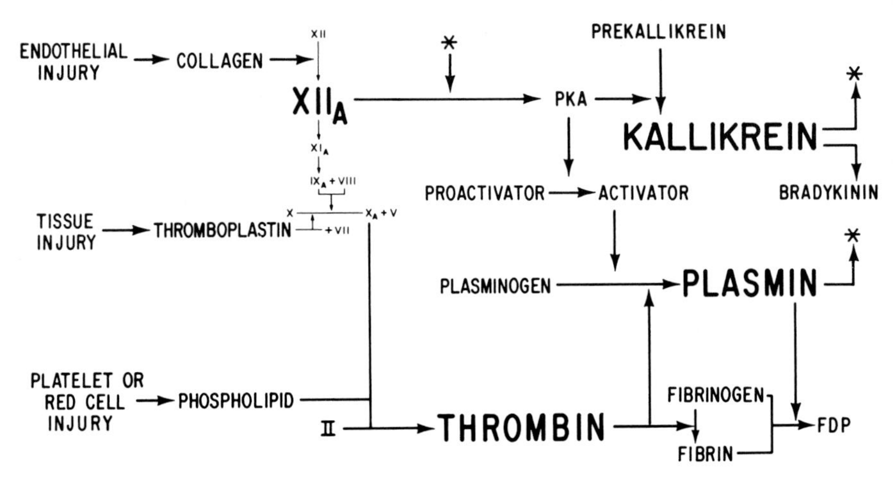

Figure I–1. Pathogenesis of DIC. (Colman, Robboy, and Minna: *Am J Med*, *52*:679, 1972).

should be stressed that in the actual clinical situation no one of these mechanisms may itself be sufficient to initiate the entire system, and positive and negative feedback mechanisms modulate the response.

Activation of Hageman factor is one possible initiating mechanism in DIC and in the induction of defensive host responses to DIC. In viremia (116), heat stroke (4,187), meningococcemia (128), gram positive endotoxemia (201) and hyperacute renal allograft rejection (28), the endothelium may be disrupted and Hageman factor activated. In gram negative septicemia with endotoxemia, necrotic endothelial cells may even detach and circulate (67).

In addition to its action on the coagulation system Hageman factor directly or indirectly activates at least three other proteolytic enzyme precursors present in plasma: prekallikrein (26,88), plasminogen (154) and complement (47) (Fig. I–1). When Hageman factor transforms plasma prekallikrein into kallikrein (143), bradykinin is released (70) and it can act as a potent vasodilator to cause hypotension (55). In hypotensive septicemia, Hageman factor activation appears to be responsible for both the initiation of coagulation (DIC) and the hypotension (via an activated kallikrein system) (128). Conversely, in the DIC associated with neoplasia, (presumably caused by the release of thromboplastin from damaged tumor cells) Hageman factor is not affected and the blood pressure remains normal and the kallikrein system stable (127). When vasoconstriction is prevented experimentally by Dibenzyline®, an alpha receptor blocker, DIC does not occur in an experimental animal model (136). The formation of kallikrein may protect the vessel where it is formed since bradykinin would antagonize any vasoconstriction (213).

Another action dependent on Hageman factor is the transformation of plasminogen into plasmin (150) which in turn initiates fibrinolysis, a physiological response to, and a finding constantly seen with DIC. If the fibrinolytic system is inhibited by epsilonaminocaproic acid (EACA), DIC is unmasked and its effects potentiated (119).

A final important consequence of Hageman factor activation is to activate the first component of the complement system

(47) in the fluid phase, thereby triggering successive steps of another proteolytic cascade. Thus, Hageman factor activates at least four proteolytic enzyme systems in the plasma and probably serves to integrate the host reaction of the inflammatory response to vessel injury (99,117).

Thromboplastic substances, which injured tissues and vessels release into the circulation, initiate the extrinsic system of blood coagulation (64) and may be a second pathway triggering DIC. Several tumors commonly associated with DIC contain more thromboplastin than most other tissues (155). High concentrations of thromboplastin and other procoagulants in leukocytes such as proteases may explain the high incidence of DIC observed in leukemia (200) and with leukemic cell destruction consequent to chemotherapy (102) (Table III-I). The hypothesis has been directly tested by infusing tissue thromboplastin and observing the initiation of DIC (64,202).

In a third possible mechanism, injured red cells (157) leukocytes and platelets (56) release phospholipids and these are postulated to accelerate blood coagulation. Examples of diseases underlying DIC which are mediated in part by ruptured erythrocytes are malaria (41), microangiopathic hemolytic anemia (14), mismatched plasma (109) or blood (99) transfusions, and experimental intravascular hemolysis (29, 107, 108).

A common feature of these hemolytic processes is the rapid, severe and intravascular nature of the red cell destruction. Most hemolytic anemias which involve extravascular destruction of red cells are not associated with clinically apparent DIC. Although it is not clear whether platelet injury alone can elicit DIC, platelets contain or have absorbed onto their surface membranes many procoagulants (factors V, VIII, XII, XIII, and phospholipids) which can be released by injury and thereby initiate DIC. In addition viruses and endotoxin directly aggregate platelets (137).

The above mechanisms all funnel through a final common pathway and result in the formation of thrombin, a proteolytic enzyme with multiple effects on coagulation proteins and platelets. The most important is the proteolytic cleavage of fibrinogen into fibrin monomer. During this process two small fibrinopeptides, A and B, are liberated; the former possesses important pharmacological properties, causing vasoconstriction of systemic (34) and pulmonary (8) vessels. Fibrin monomers spontaneously and reversibly polymerize, forming fibrin clots which are initially associated only by noncovalent bonds.

Another plasma enzyme, fibrin stabilizing factor (factor XIII) is also converted into its active form by thrombin and is requisite to form the covalent amide bonds that stabilize the fibrin clot. When factor XIII is present in low concentrations the fibrin clot appears more susceptible to fibrinolysis (74). Thrombin also irreversibly aggregates platelets at concentrations much lower than that needed to clot fibrinogen. The effect is to remove platelets from the circulation (137).

Thrombin participates in several feedback reactions. For example, thrombin can mediate platelet release of serotonin and adenosine diphosphate and increase the availability of phospholipid components (platelet factor 3) necessary for the factor IX-VIII interaction and the factor V-X complex formation (210). Thrombin also releases platelet factor 4 (57), a protein capable of neutralizing heparin, from platelets. The presence of this protein may account for the relative heparin resistance often seen during the early stages of DIC.

Thrombin increases the activity of factor V, a protein necessary for optimal thrombin formation. Thrombin altered factor V is much more unstable than native factor V and decays at a more rapid rate (25); thus, the final concentration of factor V in acute DIC is usually low. Similar mechanisms may help to explain low factor VIII levels in DIC. Finally, thrombin appears to directly activate plasminogen (54) and provides a crucial link to the fibrinolytic system. Thus, thrombin directly causes the consumption of fibrinogen, platelets, plasminogen, and factors II, V, VIII and XIII.

The fibrinolysis secondary to DIC is responsible for the hemorrhagic features frequently encountered. Damaged tissues, such as the prostate, kidney (190) and possibly red cells (183) release plasminogen activators which in turn initiate the fibrinolytic system. Plasmin destroys the same proteins that thrombin activates (fibrinogen, and factors V and VIII) and may cause platelet aggregation (148). Therefore, quantitative factor determinations may not discriminate between the roles of thrombin and plasmin.

Plasmin may be formed systemically, for example, during exercise, but is neutralized rapidly by antiplasmin and is therefore rarely observed. Yet, substantial digestion of the clot may occur, implying that significant amounts of plasmin have been generated. To solve this paradox one must consider the location of plasmin generation (gel phase vs. fluid phase). When plasminogen activators reach high levels in blood, they can penetrate any clots that are present (gel phase) and activate the adsorbed plasminogen to plasmin. Thus the clots are dissolved locally, despite the lack of free plasmin in the systemic circulation (fluid phase) (185).

The fibrinogen degradation products produced by plasmin are pivotal to the occurrence of the hemorrhagic diathesis in DIC. Since plasmin performs an extensive and continuing digestion when permitted to react with fibrinogen over long periods of time (125,126), the degradation products formed are of varied sizes and these have characteristic properties. After a short period of plasmin digestion of fibrinogen (molecular weight (MW) 320,000), fragment X (MW 240,000) is formed and is fully clottable by thrombin even though it clots more slowly than normal fibrinogen.

Fragment X is degraded further to fragment Y (MW 150,000) and fragment D (MW 83,000); neither is clottable. Fragment Y directly inhibits the action of thrombin on fibrinogen while fragment D is responsible for disordered fibrin polymerization frequently seen in DIC. Finally, the Y fragment is further degraded to form additional D fragments plus E fragments (MW 50,000) the latter having short half-disappearance times (60). Fragment E, which has little effect on coagulation, is the only degradation product excreted into the urine. The methods of determination of these polypeptides will be discussed in the next chapter.

From the foregoing summary of the pathogenesis, it is clear that nearly all the laboratory findings in DIC can be conceptualized as actions of thrombin and/or plasmin. However, many biochemical events are yet to be elucidated.

DIAGNOSIS

A major difficulty in the care of patients with DIC has been a lack of accepted criteria for diagnosis of DIC and its response to therapy. The clinical presentation of an acquired hemorrhagic-thrombotic diathesis suggests DIC. However, questions of major clinical importance remain. What laboratory tests substantiate the diagnosis of DIC with a high degree of accuracy? Are tests available that are easy to perform so that they may be used routinely in caring for critically ill patients? What are the types, frequency and mechanisms of clinical manifestations? What factors influence survival and clinical response to various therapies? Can one correlate coagulation tests, organ damage and pathological changes?

The concept of a profile of simultaneously abnormal coagulation tests and specific clotting factors in DIC has emerged in the literature. In particular the triad of prolongation of the prothrombin time, thrombocytopenia, and hypofibrinogenemia has been noted (81,82,100,116,130,177,208). Many reports suggest that FDP are also present (131,198). The clinical study on which this monograph is based represents an attempt to select patients exhibiting part or all of the above triad from a group referred to us because of an acquired bleeding or thrombotic diathesis, abnormal coagulation tests, or underlying disease frequently reported to be associated with DIC (e.g., shock, septicemia or neoplasia). The criteria we selected to diagnose DIC appear in Tables I-I and XIII-I. These criteria were formulated during the study period, and have proven useful in distinguishing between bleeding patients with and without DIC.

PATIENTS STUDIED

The 60 patients from the Massachusetts General Hospital (MGH) presented in this book were selected by prospective (Cases 1 through 45, Table I-II) and retrospective (Cases i through xv, Table XII-II) methods. A prospective search was made for patients with DIC between July 1967 and January 1970. All patients (91 in total) who were referred to the

TABLE I-I
CRITERIA FOR DIAGNOSIS OF DIC

Test	Normal value (mean ± 1 SD)	Criteria for DIC[1]	DIC % abnormal	DIC values (mean ± 1 SD)
			Screening (60 patients, 69 episodes)[3]	
Prothrombin time (sec)	12.0 ± 1.0	≥15	91%	18 (14.5 – 48)[2]
Platelets / ul	250,000 ± 50,000	≤150,000	93%	52,000 ± 48,000
Fibrinogen (mg / dl)	230 ± 35	≤160	77%	131 ± 84
			Confirmatory (45 patients, 54 episodes)[4]	
Fi titer	<1:8	≥1:16	92%	1:52 (1:11 – 1:256)[2]
Thrombin time (sec)	20 ± 1.6	≥25	59%	27 (21 – 36)[2]
Euglobulin lysis time (min)	>120	≤120	42%	

Diagnosis of DIC Requires

Abnormal screening tests	Confirmatory test	Patients[4]
3 / 3	Not required	89%
2 / 3	Required	20%
0–1 / 3	Required + fibrin thrombi	9%

[1] Values greater than 2 SD from normal mean values.
[2] Range of ± 2 SD.
[3] Prospective and retrospective studies combined. See Tables I-II and XII-II.
[4] Prospective study.

Hematology Research Laboratory for evaluation of acquired bleeding or thrombotic disorders were examined by us. Prothrombin time (PT), platelet count, fibrinogen level, tests for FDP, and other pertinent tests were performed. If abnormal titers of FDP were present or the triad of prolonged PT, thrombocytopenia and hypofibrinogenemia was present during the first week of examination, the patients were followed (45 of the 91 patients) (Tables I-II and I-III).

Five-sixths of the patients meeting the coagulation criteria had additional clinical evidence of DIC: bleeding, thrombosis or acral cyanosis. Although these clinical criteria were followed as indicators of response to therapy, they were not used in the initial selection of patients for prospective study. If the coagulation test criteria were not met, the patients were not followed at that time, but their medical records were examined retrospectively (46 of 91 patients). Three of these patients were found subsequently to have had DIC (see Table XII-II, patients i-iii).

The 45 patients with DIC were prospectively followed for bleeding (severity, number and location of sites), transfusion requirement, thrombosis, hypotension, sepsis, signs of organ dysfunction possibly related to DIC and the response of bleeding, thrombosis or acral cyanosis to therapy. Therapy for each patient was individually determined. In most instances, we gave only recommendations for diagnostic tests and therapy; the final decision always remained with the patient's primary physician. None of the 45 patients had a familial or past history of bleeding. The patients were numbered Cases 1 through 45, with letter suffixes to denote multiple episodes of DIC, e.g., Case 33A, 33B. Several case histories have been reported previously (30,90,162,173,175, 176,181,193).

All fibrinogen determinations performed by the MGH Clinical Chemistry Laboratory between November 1967 and June 1969 were reviewed (860 patients) and the patients with fibrinogen levels below 160 mg/dl (greater than 2 standard deviations below the normal mean value (230 mg/dl) for the laboratory) were ascertained (retrospective study). Patients on cardiopulmonary bypass, patients with severe liver disease

TABLE I-II
CLINICAL AND LABORATORY FINDINGS IN 45 PATIENTS WITH DIC

			ETIOLOGY		PRESENTATION				CLINICAL BLEEDI					
Case #	MGH UNIT #	Sex and Age	Primary Disease	Additional Factors Precipitating or Predisposing Patient to DIC	Hypotension	Mode of Presentation	Duration of Bleeding	Combined Scoring of Severity of bleeding	# Bleeding Sites	Purpura, petechiae (P = palpable purpura)	Wound, Venapuncture	Mucosal	Hematoma	G
1	MB 1533071	58 F	Serratia Septicemia	Hypoxemia Acidosis	+	Sudden bleed.	A	Sevr	5		+	+	+	-
2	BI 0870632	80 M	Acute Myelo-monocytic Leuk		–	Hematem-isis			3	+	+			
3	JC 1540052	16 F	N meningiditis septicemia		+	Purpura Meningit	A	Mod	4	P		+		
4	KO 1536669	3d F	Aortic Coarctation	Hepatic conges Acidosis	–	GI bleed	A	Sevr	5					+
5A	MS 1441376	40 M	Acute Promye-locytic Leuk	VAMP chemoRx	–	Lab (screen)	A	Mod	1		+			
5B				ChemoRx	–	Diffuse bleed	A	Sevr	7	+	+	+	+	+
6A	HV 0570226	74 M	Purp fulminans β Streptococcal	Allergic drug reaction, Post-		Diffuse ecchymo	6w	Mod	5	P			+	
6B			infect. throat, skin	necrotic cirrhosis	+	Purpura	A	Mod	2	P			+	
7	HM 1329467	54 M	Bleeding Duodenal ulcer	EACA Rx, Vascular Surg.	+	Diffuse bleed	A	Sevr	4		+	+		+
8A	BV 0808902	55 M	Carcinoma lung	Hypoxia	–	Purpura	4w	Mild	3	+				+
8B				Arteriotomy	+	Stroke Syndrome	A	None	0					
9	MM 1587187	8 M	Acute Lympho-blastic Leuk.	L-aspariginase chemoRx	=	Lab (Fi,fib)		None	0					
10A	ER 1478835	32 M	Cirrhosis N mening		–	Diffuse purpura	A	Mod	2	P				
10B			Septicemia	EACA Rx	–	Lab (screen)	None		0					
11	ES 1598366	21 F	N gonorrhoeae septicemia		–	Erythema nodules	None		0					
12	DC 1082555	61 M	Ca Prostate	P32 chemoRx	+	Diffuse bleed	A	Sevr	8	+	+	+		+
13A	WK 1100802	66 M	Ca prostate		–	Hemar-throsis	4w	Mild	3	+				
13B				Estrogen Rx	–	Purpura Hematuria	A	Mild	3		+		+	
14	MG 1533924	24 F	N meningiditis septicemia		+	Purpura	A	Mod	1	P				
15	EV 1547099	61 F	Aortic aneurysm	EACA Rx Cardiac pump	+	Massive bleed	A	Serv	5		+			
16A	CU 1486951	50 M	Acute Promyelocytic	ChemoRx (Ara-C)		Massive bleed	A	Mod	4	+		+		+
16B			Leukemia	ChemoRx		Hematoma	A	Sevr	3				+	+
16C			Klebsiella Septicemia	ChemoRx	+	Hemoptys Hematoma	A	Sevr	4	P			+	
17	EM 1540150	9 F	Meningitis (?aseptic)	Transfusion re-action acidosis	+	Petech	A	Mod	3	+				+
18	MS 0979364	74 M	Ca prostate		–	Diffuse bleed	A	Mild	3	+				+
19	FB 0871969	75 F	Dissect aortic aneurysm	Cardiac arrest	+	Diffuse bleed	A	Mild	4	+	+		+	
20	KC 1486445	24 F	N meningiditis septicemia	Pregnant	+	Diffuse Purpura	A	Mod	6	P	+			+

			LABORATORY											OUTCOME	FIBRIN THROMBI
			ROUTINE			SCREENING		CONFIRMATORY			ANCILLARY				
GU	Thrombi clinically	Miscellaneous (Bleeding Sites) [Thrombotic sites]	Hematocrit	WBC (1000/μl)	Reticulocyte count (%)	Prothrombin Time (sec)	Platelet count (1000/μl)	Fibrinogen (mg/dl)	Fi titer	ELT (min)	Thrombin Time (sec)	Plasminogen (units/ml)	PTT (sec)	Length of Survival from onset of Symptomatic DIC	[Autopsy] (Biopsy)
			18	29	2.0	17	9	108	1:16(SC)	nl	27	1.4	49	d 4 days	
			18	197		25	59	40	1:160	Immed	35	1.9		d 3 hr	
			34	35		16	77	310	1:10	nl	85			alive	(+)
		(Pulm,CNS)	32	24	3.9	27	24	96	1:40	nl	39		120	d 4 days	[+]
			15	71	0.2	20	75	50			90		nl	d 17 days	
+		(Eye) (Pulm)	18	136	0.3	19	32	264						d 2 days	[+]
	+	Escars (Trunk)	28	23		27	52	86	1:80[1]	nl[1]			64	d 8 days	
	+	Escars (Scalp)	26	13	5.9	17	160	140					55	d 1 day	[+]
+			24	13	4.6	25	50	142	1:10	nl	31			d 5 days	
	+	[Super.VV]	23	72	6.8	21	52	138	1:10[1]	nl[1]	23[1]			d 45 days	[+]
	+	(Pleurol) [CNS]	28	39	0.9	26	15	42						d 1 day	[+]
			26	7	0.9	13	110	170	1:32					alive	
+			37	5	3.6	24	46	200			28		59		(−)
			35	6	4.2	27	46	138	1:10	nl				d 8 months	[−]
			44	13		13	214		1:16				24	alive	
+		(Pulm)	35	42	1.3	22	29	60	1:160	nl[1]				d 2 days	[+]
+		(Epistax (Hemar-throsis	34	7		18	65	74	1:1280	10	25	2.3	45		
+			32	8		20	34	94	1:2560	90		2.6	53	alive	
		Acrocy	27	25	1.3	15	56	324	1:10	nl		2.3	39	alive	
	+	[Spinal cord]	32	19		16	180	350	1:16	5	23	3.4	36	d 9 days	[+]
+		(Pulm)	26	4		22	18	100				1.5	91	d 30 days	
		(Epistax)	15	1	1.7	26	14	42	1:10	120	25			d 12 days	
		(Pulm, CNS)	24			26	18	70						d 1 day	[+]
		(Eye)	29	10	0.6	24	3	100	1:160	nl				alive	
+			33	14		19	26	130		nl	25		nl	d 14 days	[−]
			27	6	2.7	15	55	110		nl	25			d 17 days	[+]
+		(Vaginal) (Pleural)	45	16		109	68	NC	1:512	Immed	NC		NC	d 4 hr.	[+]

TABLE I-11 (Continued)
CLINICAL AND LABORATORY FINDINGS IN 45 PATIENTS WITH DIC

	ETIOLOGY								CLINICAL					
					PRESENTATION						BLEEDI			
Case #	MGH UNIT #	Sex and Age	Primary Disease	Additional Factors Precipitating or Predisposing Patient to DIC	Hypotension	Mode of Presentation	Duration of Bleeding	Combined Scoring of Severity of bleeding	# Bleeding Sites	Purpura, petechiae (P = palpable purpura)	Wound, Venapuncture	Mucosal	Hematoma	
21	GF 1491911	33 M	Acute Promyelocytic Leukemia	Transfusion reaction	–	Purpura Epistax	3w	Mod	5	+	+	+		
22	JC 1616732	6d M	E. coli septicemia	PO Hirschprung Resp arrest	–	Lab (plt)	None		0					
23	NW 1425671	68 M	Ca prostate		–	Hematuria	1 yr	Mild	1					
24	FD 1306337	68 M	Ca prostate		–	Hematoma	A	Mod	3	+	+		+	
25	SW 0979825	45 F	S aureus pneumonia	Barbit ingest Hypoxia	+	Hematoma	A	Mild	3	+	+		+	
26	BD 1546019	39 F	N meningiditis septicemia		+	Purpura	A	Mod	3	P				+
27	MB 0470144	55 F	Acute Myelo-Monocytic Leuk	ChemoRx (6-MP,Ara-C)	–	Hemoptys Purpura	A	Mild	4	+	+			+
28	CT 1607583	66 M	Aspergillus septicemia		–	Purpura	3w	Sevr	9	+	+		+	+
29	JN 1556499	46 F	Acute myelomonocytic Leuk	ChemoRx (6 MP)		Purpura Vag bld	A	Mod	2	+				
30	LD 1554876	17 F	Cardiac arrest PO abortion	Acidosis	+	Vag, GI Hematur	A	Mod	3					+
31	JB 1556398	32 F	P pneumoniae septicemia		+	Acrocy	A	Mild	3	P				
32	PM 0916531	49 M	Gram reg pneumonia	Acidosis Hypoxia		GI,wound bleed	A A	Mild Mild	5 5	+ +	+			+
33A	MC 1563186	18 M	Viral myocarditis & pneumonitis		+	Venapunc bleed	A	Mild	3		+			+
33B				Amputate arm Hypoxia,Acidosis	+	Acrocy Petech	A	Mild	4	+	+	+		
34	CG 0810496	66 M	Hemolyt anemia Coombs pos	Pneumothorax	+	Lab (screen)	A	Sevr	5		+			
35A	BW 0235736	69 F	Hypotension	Duodenal ulcer Post hepatitis	+	Hematem	A	Sevr	4		+		+	+
35B			S albus endocarditis		+	Petech	A	Sevr	2	+				+
36	EC 1542938	81 M	Klebsiella septicemia		+	Acrocy	None		0					
37	AD 1514861	60 M	Streptococcal septicemia	Cirrhosis	–	Diffuse bleed	A	Sevr	6	+	+	+		+
38	LA 1607642	53 M	P aerguinosa septicemia	Acute MI Cardiac arrest	+	GI bleed Hematoma	A	Mild	4	+	+		+	+
39	JS 1575012	41 F	Acute myelogenous Leuk	ChemoRx (6TG,Ara-C)	–	Lab (screen)	None		0					
40	AF 0084164	69 F	Hepatitis fulminant	Cardiac arrest P.mirabilis sept	+	Diffuse bleed	A	Sevr	6	+		+		+
41	JF 1082087	77 M	Streptococcal peritonitis	? amyloidosis	+	Lab (screen)	A	Mod	5			+		+
42	FC 1615353	13 M	N meningiditis septicemia		–	Purpura	A	Mod	2	+				+
43	RZ 1615586	51 F	S aureus pneumonia	Hypoxia	+	Acrocy	A	Mild	2	+				+
44	MD 0879409	74 F	Salmonella septicemia		+	Hematoma	A	Mod	1		+ +		+ +	
45	DL 1027505	15 F	Aspergillus septicemia	Chronic Active Hepatitis	–	Purpura	A	Sevr	6	+	+	+	+	+

		LABORATORY ROUTINE SCREENING					CONFIRMATORY				ANCILLARY		OUTCOME	FIBRIN THROMBI
Thrombi clinically	Miscellaneous (Bleeding Sites) [Thrombotic sites]	Hematocrit	WBC (1000/μl)	Reticulocyte count (%)	Prothrombin Time (sec)	Platelet count (1000/μl)	Fibrinogen (mg/dl)	Fi titer	ELT (min)	Thrombin Time (sec)	Plasminogen (units/ml)	PTT (sec)	Length of Survival from onset of Symptomatic DIC	[Autopsy] (Biopsy)
	(Epistax)	15	12		25	19	160	1:80	Immed				d 6 days	[+]
	(Eye,CNS)	31	5			9	100	1:64					d 7days	[+]
		31	14	4.1	18	83	220		30	24		65	d 3 months	
	(Pulm)	32	16		47	147	240	1:128	Immed		1.9	80	alive	
		29	16	1.4	18	10	124	1:512	nl			46	d 1 day	
	(Acral G vaginal)	23	23	2.4	20	33	133	1:512	nl				alive	
	(Pulm)	31	12	0.8	17	7	96	1:32 (TRCHII)	nl	21	5.0	26	d 5 days	
	(Epistax) (Hemoptys)	23	10	9.8	17	6	70	1:32	nl	32		26	d 10 days	[+]
	(Vaginal) (Pulm)	22	115	0.4	15	19	110	1:8	95	24	2.7	25	d 36 days	
	(Vaginal)	23	19		28	129	167	1:512		55			alive	
	Acrocy [Acral Gangrene]	43	73	2.0	14	51	240	1:256	Immed nl	22	0.5	34	alive	(+)
		32	11		17	15	110	1:32		15		80	d 4 day	[+]
	[Gangrene [limb]	30	36		31	14	96	1:256	Immed 3		1.4		d 9 days	
	Acrocy	37	53		17	25	168				1.1	53	d 1 day	[+]
		30	33	6.0	16	18	97	1:2	nl	26		48	d 7 days	
	Acrocy	27	13	6.0	16	27	96	1:32	nl	24		42	d 13 days	
		28	9		25	20	34	1:128	15	37	3.5	41	d 2 days	[+]
	[Acral +Gangrene]	32	11	3.2	18	144	340	1:32					alive	
	(Pleural)	34	6		25	91	60	1:64	55	27		58	d 4 days	
		37	23		25	65	200	1:32	nl	23		24	d 2 days	[+]
		23	24	1.0	14	21	96	1:32	nl	24			d 30 days	[+]
	(Vaginal)	38	10	3.2	43	12	60	1:16	5	34	1.7	50	d 1 day	[+]
	(Epistax) (Tracheal)	27	25	1.6	19	15	156	1:16	nl	27			d 2 day	
		45	97		55	57	NC	1:128				80	d 1 hr	[+]
+	[Acral Gangrene]	31	4	0.6	24	90	140	1:16	nl	35		120	d 5 days	[+]
		29	12	1.0	17	78	117	1:16		21		34	d 3 months	
	(Vaginal) (Eye,Pulm)	30	21	1.4	26	13	110	1:16		33		52	d 5 days	[+]

TABLE I-III

CHANGE IN COAGULATION TESTS ASSOCIATED WITH THE DEVELOPMENT AND TREATMENT OF DIC

CASE #	DEVELOPMENT OF DIC (NET CHANGE)				THERAPY								INTERVAL TO RESPONSE	RESPONSE TO THERAPY OF DIC (NET CHANGE)						
	Δ HCT	Δ PT (sec)	Δ PLATELETS (1000 / μl)	Δ FIBRINOGEN (mg / dl)	HEPARIN (USP UNITS[1] iv q 4 h)	BLOOD—PLASMA (units)	PLATELETS (units)	FIBRINOGEN (gm)	VITAMIN K	PRESSOR AGENTS	CORTICOSTEROIDS	ANTIBIOTICS[2]	DAYS	Δ PT (sec)	Δ PLATELETS (1000 / μl)	Δ FIBRINOGEN (mg / dl)	Δ FI TITER[3] (log, base 2)	ELT[3]	BLEEDING[4] (physical exam)	COMBINED CRITERIA[5] (TABLE XI-1)
1	−17	+4	−127	−102	H (6250)	4	6	6	+			CK	4	+3	+4	+92			S	IP
2	−11	+3	−182	−350	H (2500)	8							T<0.5						NC	IND
3	− 8				H (6250)	5						P	2	−4	+14	+180	nl	nl	S	I
4	−15					2	1		+			PK	5	−12	−32	0	+1		W	W
5A	−10	+13	− 25	− 70	H (9400),E	5		5			+		9	−9	−17	+396		nl	S	*I*
5B	−13	+4	−108	−196		7					+	P	3	+4	−43	−56			W	W
6A	− 2				H (7500)	5		4	+			P	4	−12	+186	+204			S	I
6B	0	+2	−130	−150	H (11,300)	0						P	1						W	IND
7	−11				E	14			+		+	T	2	−5	−106	+110			W	W
8A						3			+			PC	10	−2	+27	+102				W
8B	−10	+8	− 64	−198		3						PC	<1						NC	IND
9	−10					0							7		+240		−4		NB	NB
10A	0				H (6250),E	0			+				2	−5	+66	+50			S	IP
10B	− 3	+7	−134	−82	E→H (6250)	0						P	7	−5	+121	+88			NB	NB
11	0					0						P	?						NB	NB
12	−13	+10	−300		H (6250),E	4		4	+		+		1	−4	+14	+214			P	IP
13A	0				H (6250)	0							2	−3	+22	+112	−1	nl	S	I
13B	− 3	+5	−32	−108	H (9400)	0							8	−7	+25	+126	−10	nl	S	I
14	− 8				H (3120)	6						P	1	−4	+27	+98	−2	nl	S	I
15	0	+4	−517		E	15						OS	1	−3	−115	+40		nl	S	W
16A	− 8	+6	−13	−200	H (6250)	3					+	PC	4	−5	+7	+134			P	IP
16B	−15	+10	−5	−138		10					+	O	[illegible]	−9	0	+188			P	IP

16C	−11	+10	+10	−150	H (6250)	6				+	C	1	−9	−15	+90			W	IND
17	− 4				H (3120)	3	13			+	PSu	4		+41	+200	+3		W	W
18	0					1						3	−3	+72				W	W
19	− 7					5						2	+1	+74	+88			S	I
20	0				H (6250)	1		+	+	+		T<0.5						NC	IND
21	− 2				H (7500),E	3					P	5	−6	−12	+80			P	IP
22	0		−269		H (3120)	3					GC	3		+5		−4		NB	NB
23	0	+4	−119	−130	E	0				+	A	4						S	IP
24	−11				H (9400)	12						2	−31	+7	+370	−3	nl	S	I
25	− 1		−200	−192		1					OC	1						NC	IND
26	−20				H (3120)	0		+	+		P	2	−7	−9	+357			S	I
27	− 7	+5	−15	−376	H (6250)	0		+		+		2	−1	−2	+192			NC	U
28					H (6250)	15	3			+		1+	−4	+16	+40			P	IP
29	0				H (5000)	4	14			+		7	−2	+6	+180			S	I
30	−12					6			+			2	−16	−8	+73	−5	nl	S	I
31	0				H (5000)	0				+	PCO	4	+1	+331	+440	−4		S	I
32	0		−130	−650	H (9400)	3						4	−3	+165	+60	−3		S	I
33A	− 8	+18	−209	−312	H (3120)	2		+	+	+		1	−12	+44	+40	−2	Improv	S	I
33B	− 3	+2	−96	−85	H (3120)	1			+		CGCe	0.5	−1	−2	+28			NC	IND
34	0	+2	−326			0				+	T	2	−1	−2	+21			W	W
35A	−18	+4	−169	−184	H (5000)	6		+		+		1	−3	+5	+168	−2		S	I
35B	−18	+7		−230	H (6250),E	6				+	O	2	+5	+10	+66	−1	Worse	W	W
36	− 8	+3	−78	−640	H (6250)	5			+		PKC	4	−3	+419	+280			NB,A	I
37	− 3	+2	−85		H (5000)	11		+			P	4	−3	−19	+60	−3	nl	P	IP
38	− 6	+10	−195	−440	H (5000)	0						1	−7	+45	+60			S	I
39	−13	+2	−174	−244		0						4	−1	−6	+144	−4		NB	NB
40	− 4	+24	−193			7		+		+		1	−20		+20			NC	IND
41	−11	+6	−216	−214	H (6250)	0		+	+	+	PN	3						NC	U
42	0				H (6250)	0					PA	<1						NC	IND
43	−14	+11	−96	−260	H (9400)	7			+		KOGC	4	−5	+95	+330	−3		P	IP
44	−13					9			+		PC	2	−4	+22	+123			S	I
45	− 7	+4	−76	−70		8		+		+	CCe							W	W

[1] Therapy: H, heparin; E, epsilon aminocaproic acid at i.v. dose of 1 g per hour.

[2] Antibiotics: A, ampicillin; C, chloramphenicol; Ce, cephalin; G, gentamicin; K, kanamycin; N, neomycin; O, oxacillin; P, penicillin; S, streptomycin; Su, sulfasoxazole; T, tetracycline.

[3] NL, ELT or Fi titer becomes normal from an abnormal value.

[4] Bleeding: NB, no bleeding; NC, no change; P, partially stops bleeding (all major bleeding stops); S, all bleeding stops; W, bleeding worse.

[5] See Table XI-I for combined clinical and coagulation criteria. I, improves completely; IP, improves partially; IND, indeterminate; U, unchanged; W, worse.

whose fibrinogen level was above 125 mg/dl (see Table XIII-I), and patients already in the prospective study were excluded. The remaining all had a prolonged PT and thrombocytopenia in addition to hypofibrinogenemia. These patients are presented as a retrospective study (Table XII-II, cases iv-xv).

CHAPTER II

THE LABORATORY DIAGNOSIS OF DIC

WHEN BLEEDING AND/OR THROMBOSIS occur in a patient where there is a clinical setting known to predispose to DIC, coagulation tests that are capable of reflecting abnormalities in the hemostatic mechanism can be used to confirm or eliminate the diagnosis. The activation or action of thrombin directly causes consumption of fibrinogen, factors II, V, VIII and XIII, platelets and plasminogen. *In vivo,* but not *in vitro,* factors XII, XI, IX and X may also be decreased due to the formation of activated intermediates and their subsequent removal by the reticuloendothelial system or by other metabolic activities of the liver. In addition, the secondary activation of the fibrinolytic system results in the formation of FDP which interfere with the formation of fibrin by the action of thrombin (see Chapter I).

The following sections are detailed descriptions of the coagulation tests used in this study. Problems of interpretation are included for reference.

SCREENING TESTS

There is no single test pathognomic of DIC. Because of the need for rapid diagnosis in a seriously bleeding patient, criteria were selected that relied principally on laboratory tests available in most hematologic departments. The one-stage PT (165), fibrinogen determination as clottable protein (169) and platelet count (Coulter Counter, Model B), all of which were performed on fresh specimens (average of 12 times per patient on separate days), are available on a 24-hour basis in most medical centers.

Prothrombin Time (PT)

The prothrombin time is the clotting time obtained by adding an excess of a potent thromboplastin reagent and an optimal amount of calcium to plasma under standardized conditions. This test measures factors I, II, V, VII and X (extrinsic coagulation system). The PT is prolonged only when the concentration of any single factor is below a certain critical level or when a circulating anticoagulant, e.g., FDP or heparin, is present. Since the normal clotting time of the PT is about 12 seconds, more thrombin is formed than is utilized in the thrombin time (*vide infra*) in which the control is set at 20 ± 1 second. Thus the PT is less sensitive to heparin or FDP than the thrombin time. Familial studies of congenital hypofibrinogenemia suggest that fibrinogen levels greater than 100 mg/dl do not affect the PT and that at levels of about 75 mg/dl the PT is not more than 2 sec prolonged (83,218) (which is still 1 sec less than our criteria of an abnormal PT of 3 sec prolongation). Congenital deficiencies of other clotting factors suggest that the critical levels which will prolong the PT are: Factor V, 55% = 1 sec (133); Factor VII, < 30% = 1–4 sec (45); Factor X, 70% = 1 sec, < 50% = > 2 sec (75,178). Factor II (true prothrombin) must be reduced to 25% or less before the PT is prolonged more than 2 sec. Thus the PT reflects well the decrease in II, V and X usually seen in DIC.

For calculations the percent PT is determined according to Quick (165) where 12 sec = 100% and 21 sec = 10%.

Fibrinogen

The fibrinogen level in plasma is determined by the conversion of fibrinogen to fibrin after the enzyme thrombin is added exogenously (169). The fibrin is then removed from the solution and quantified by the biuret reaction (40). This method measures only clottable protein and is unlike salting-out methods which measure fibrin, non-clottable fibrinogen derivatives, and other plasma globulins of similar solubilities

(78). In a normal patient true fibrinogen is the only clottable protein. In DIC, small to large amounts of FDP or fibrin complexes are also clottable and therefore are also measured. At very high levels of FDP, no fibrin may form due to complete inhibition of thrombin action by these products.

Platelet Count

The platelet count (determined by phase contrast microscopy or the Coulter Counter method) must be evaluated in light of other underlying causes for its depression. Bone marrow examination is frequently of great help (see Chap. VII).

CONFIRMATORY TESTS

Abnormalities in all three of the screening tests confirm the diagnosis of DIC. If any one is normal, confirmatory tests must be used. Confirmatory tests performed in our laboratory include euglobulin clot lysis time (ELT) (97), thrombin time (TT) (199), Fi test (198), staphylococcal clumping tests (SCT) (84), Thrombo-Wellco test (53) and tanned red cell hemagglutination inhibition test (TRCHII) (131).

Thrombin Time (TT)

The simplest and most suitable test for routine confirmation is the thrombin time which is the clotting time resulting when a standard amount of exogenous thrombin is added to plasma. A control reaction is constructed in which a solution of purified thrombin in a calcium containing buffer will clot fresh normal plasma in about 20 seconds (199). This thrombin solution is then added to the test plasma and the clotting time noted. The thrombin time is prolonged in the presence of FDP, heparin, or markedly decreased fibrinogen levels. Prolongation of five or more seconds (> 3 standard deviations) beyond control values is abnormal in this study. By this definition, a level of fibrinogen of 75 mg/dl or more will not in itself result in an abnormal thrombin time (Table XII-III)

(86). If the thrombin time is used as one of the initial battery of tests (prior to heparin therapy), an abnormal result almost always signifies the presence of FDP, or severe hypofibrinogenemia, both indicative of DIC.

For calculations the units TT are determined according to Biggs and MacFarland (9) where 20 sec = 2.0 units and 40 sec = 1.0 units.

Euglobulin Clot Lysis Time (ELT)

The ELT measures plasmin and/or plasminogen activators after the removal of inhibitors (97). We consider a lysis time of 120 minutes or less as abnormal and interpret it as reflecting increased levels of plasminogen activators, or plasmin. In this test the euglobulin fraction is precipitated and contains nearly all the plasminogen, plasminogen activator, and about 20 percent of the fibrinogen of the parent plasma; the plasmin inhibitors remain largely in the supernatant (97).

Even though the ELT is simple to perform and useful in diagnosis, numerous technical and theoretical problems are known. For example, studies (22) have shown that the temperature at which the test is run and the time lapse after which the sample is collected are critical factors in the preservation of the labile activator substance. Others have suggested that pH is also critical (85) and determines the amount of plasminogen and plasmin precipitated in the euglobulin fraction. A more serious consideration concerns the theoretical effect of low levels of fibrinogen. However, our data (Chapters V and XII) and that of others (129) suggest that hypofibrinogenemia alone will not result in an abnormal ELT. A decrease in plasminogen as occurs in fibrinolysis may result in a prolonged ELT. The ELT may not accurately reflect the efficacy of EACA therapy in controlling severe fibrinolysis. When the euglobulin fraction is precipitated, EACA remains in the supernatant. Thus, the *in vitro* test may not reflect the true *in vivo* state of inhibited fibrinolysis (89). Local fibrinolysis may elevate FDP without changing the euglobulin lysis time. Finally short euglobulin lysis times have been noted in apparently normal patients (97).

Fibrin Degradation Products (FDP)

By far the most sensitive tests for fibrinolysis measure the levels of FDP. Serum is collected by clotting plasma with an excess of exogenous thrombin (thereby removing *all* clottable protein) while ongoing fibrinolysis is inhibited by the addition of EACA. Residual fibrinogen-related antigen can be detected by immunodiffusion (sensitivity 40 ug/ml) or by the Fi test or TRCHII.

With the Fi test, FDP react with latex particles coated with anti-human fibrinogen (Fi reagent), producing macroscopically visible aggregates (198). Several dilutions of serum allow for quantification of the antigen. The Fi test reacts only with the fibrin monomer portions of the circulating (soluble and non-clottable) fibrin monomer-FDP complex (149) and not with fragments X or Y (the high molecular weight FDP) or fragments D or E (the low molecular weight FDP). Thus certain classes of FDP are not detected by the Fi test. An Fi titer of 1:16 or greater is considered positive. The average titer in normal subjects is 1:2 (range 0 to 1:6), (198). The sensitivity of this assay expressed as micrograms of fibrinogen equivalents per milliliter is 1.0 to 2.5 ug. Calculations are performed using the exponent to the base 2 of the Fi titer.*

The SCT measures the ability of fibrinogen and its derivatives to clump certain strains of staphylococci (84). A titer of 1:16 or greater is abnormal. The test measures complexes of X and Y but does not sensitively measure D or E. The sensitivity is 0.3–1.2 ug of fibrinogen-related antigen/ml.

The TRCHII test measures the ability of fibrinogen-related antigen to prevent the agglutination of red cells coated with fibrinogen to antihuman fibrinogen antibody (131). The test measures the late FDP, D and E, almost as well as X and

* Soon after the completion of our study, the manufacturer (Hyland Laboratories) changed from rabbit to goat antifibrinogen antibody, resulting in a much less sensitive Fi test. The differences between our sensitivity figures for the Fi test (1–2 ug/ml of fibrinogen equivalents) and that of Marder *et al.* (124) (10 ug/ml) may be due to different antisera or changes in methodology; their end point is read at 30 seconds while ours is read at 3 minutes. At the present time we use the SCT test (84) and the Thrombo-Wellco test (53), which is a latex coated particle coated with antibody to FDP D and E.

Y but is relatively insensitive to complexes (unpublished results). A titer of 1:8 or greater is abnormal. Normal individuals have less than 10 ug/ml. The sensitivity of the assay is 0.5–1.0 ug fibrinogen antigen/ml.*

New methods of measuring FDP are under evaluation. Counter-immuno electrophoresis appears relatively insensitive. The development of a radial immunodiffusion test to measure D antigen is also imminent. Agarose gel filtration of plasma combined with a sensitive method of measuring fibrinogen quantifies not only FDP but also complexes; the test, however, is time consuming and not suitable for a clinical laboratory. Paracoagulation tests with ethanol or protamine sulfate are simple to perform (148) but are relatively insensitive (200 and 40 ug fibrinogen equivalents/ml, respectively) (unpublished data) and difficult to quantify. The clinical results with such tests have been reviewed recently by Niewiarowski (148). A major problem has been the inability to quantify these tests.

OTHER TESTS

The plasminogen level measures the precursor of plasmin and is decreased when it is converted to the active enzyme. A fall of plasminogen may be due to ongoing fibrinolysis or decreased synthesis, as in liver disease. To measure plasminogen, casein hydrolysis by plasmin is quantified after plasma plasminogen has been activated by streptokinase. Normal plasminogen (3) levels for this laboratory are 5.5 ± 1.8 casein units/ml.

The whole blood clotting time (CT, normal 4–12 min, therapeutic 16–24 min) and the partial thromboplastin time (PTT, normal 22–37 sec) are well known methods (35). The PTT, although useful in diagnosis, is sensitive to heparin and cannot discriminate between decreased clotting factors and the effects of heparin during therapy (*see* "Heparin Therapy" in Chapter XI).

* The results of studies comparing the above techniques for evaluating FDP show that the Fi test, TRCHII, SCT and Thrombo-Wellco test are generally equivalent, while the immuno diffusion technique is insensitive (53,84). The correlation coefficients of the Fi test with the TRCHII and SCT are r = 0.90 and r = 0.78 respectively (Table II-I), while that of the SCT and Thrombo-Wellco test are r = 0.82.

TABLE II-I

CORRELATION OF THREE TESTS FOR DETECTING FDP[1]

Reciprocial of Titer

Case #	Fi	Staph. Clumping	TRCHII
1	1	16	8
27	2	4	32
15	16	16	8
40	16	64	64
33	64	64	64
26	64	256	256
2	128	128	64
31	256	256	128
30	512	256	128
25	512	512	256

[1] From Ref. 198. Correlation coefficients were: r = 0.90, Fi with TRCHII; and 4 = 0.78, Fi with SC.

Activation of the kallikrein system can be detected using assays for free esterase activity, prekallikrein and kallikrein inhibitor based on the hydrolysis of tosyl arginine methyl ester (TAME) (31,128). When the free esterase activity is increased, its substrate specificity must be compared to purified human kallikrein. Hageman factor (Factor XII) is assayed by a modification of the PTT using congenitally deficient plasma. However, all the tests discussed in this paragraph are complicated and restricted to use in research laboratories.

The use of clotting factor assays for diagnosis may prove confusing. Factors V, VIII, and X are frequently reduced in DIC; however, they may be normal. Factors V and VIII may be increased due to endotoxin; a normal level may represent a decrease from a previously elevated value. Also the results may vary enormously depending upon whether one or two stage methods are used (146). Our most serious criticism against using factor assays (other than fibrinogen) are the complexity of the assays, the need for specially trained technicians, the fact that these tests are not routine procedures in most hospitals, and that they are abnormal in fewer cases than the tests we have chosen.

Fibrinogen and platelet survival have shed light on the pathogenic mechanisms of DIC but are useful only as research tools at present.

CHAPTER III

CONDITIONS INITIATING OR PREDISPOSING PATIENTS TO DIC

DIC, LIKE FEVER, ANEMIA OR congestive heart failure is a symptom of a disease process that may have many different etiologies. It does not appear to be a disease in itself. Since the central principle of therapy is the correction of all underlying causes of DIC, it is important to detect all of the factors that initiate, predispose or maintain DIC in each individual patient.

The etiologic classification of DIC presented in Table III-I is based upon our conception of its pathogenesis (Fig. I-1). The major categories represent the mechanisms which probably initiate blood coagulation: a) endothelial injury; b) tissue injury; c) platelet or red cell injury; d) reticuloendothelial system injury; and e) uncertain. Within these major subdivisions only common or general disease categories are listed. Clinically this appears to be more useful than extensive listing of all possible underlying diseases that have been linked to DIC (5,186).

Each of our 60 patients (Table III-I) in the prospective (Table I-II) and retrospective (Table XII-II) studies had an underlying disorder initiating DIC. Often multiple factors appeared to be involved. The common primary conditions underlying DIC are septicemia (particularly gram negative septicemia (62,164), e.g. menigococcemia or *E. coli*—see history of Case 22), neoplasia (particularly prostatic carcinoma and acute granulocytic leukemia—see histories of Cases 5 and 39, complications of pregnancy (abruptio placenta, retained dead fetus, and amniotic fluid embolism), and prolonged severe hypotension of any etiology (*see* history of Case 35).

CASE 5—ACUTE PROMYELOCYTIC LEUKEMIA: A 40 year old black man entered for persistent bleeding after dental extraction. The

TABLE III-I

ETIOLOGICAL CLASSIFICATION OF DIC AT THE MASSACHUSETTS GENERAL HOSPITAL (PROSPECTIVE AND RETROSPECTIVE STUDY)
July 1967 - January 1970

Etiologic Class	*Number of Patients*	
	Primary disease or event	Additional factors precipitating or predisposing patient to DIC
Tissue injury (thromboplastin release)		
Obstetrical, pregnancy	1	3
Surgical	1	1
Neoplastic		
Carcinoma		
adenocarcinoma prostate	5	0
other	2	0
Leukemia		
acute granulocytic	8	0
other	1	0
Lymphoma	2	0
Associated with chemotherapy	0	13
Endothelial injury (Hageman factor activation)		
Gram negative septicemia (endotoxemia)		
Neisseria meningitidis	6	0
Other	9	4
Gram positive septicemia	8	1
Viremia	2	0
Large vessel catheterization, or surgery	0	9
Platelet or red cell injury (phospholipid release)		
Immunologic, purpura fulminans	1	1
Hemolysis		
Aspergillus	2	0
Other	2	1
Reticuloendothelial system injury		
Liver injury	3	6
Splenectomy	0	3
Uncertain		
Prolonged hypotension	3	23
Acidosis	0	9
Hypoxemia	2	9
Pancreatitis	1	0
Massive pulmonary embolism	1	0
Total	60	83

hematocrit was 20%, WBC 71,000 with 11% neutrophils, 2% band forms, 3% metamyelocytes, 12% myelocytes, 45% promyelocytes, 12% blast forms, 6% young monocytes and 9% lymphocytes. The platelet count was 101,000/ul, PT 17 sec, PTT 46 sec, bleeding time 11 min, fibrinogen 120 mg/dl and TT normal. The bone marrow was packed with myeloblasts and promyelocytes.

Therapy with transfusion, vincristine, methotrexate, 6 mercaptopurine, prednisone (VAMP) and allopurinol was begun. Two days later the platelet count fell to 76,000/ul and the fibrinogen to 50 mg/dl, while the bleeding time was 60 min, and PT 20 sec. The whole blood clot lysed in less than 2 hr and the ELT was 90 min. Factor II, V, and X were 45%, 78% and 176% of normal, respectively. Therapy with heparin (6,000 U every 6 hr) was begun. Eight hours later bleeding from a tooth socket increased and EACA (1 gm IV hourly) was added to the regimen. Shortly thereafter, large painful hematomata appeared in the antecubital fossa and buttock at venipuncture and injection sites. The fibrinogen dropped to 24 mg/dl and the PT rose to 23 sec. Because of upper and lower gastrointestinal bleeding, fresh whole blood and fibrinogen (8 gm) were given, and the heparin was increased to 9,000 U every 6 hr. By the sixth day the PT, fibrinogen, TT, ELT and Fi were normal.

During the next day, VAMP therapy was stopped when new hematomata appeared at injection sites and old hematomata enlarged. Subsequently, bleeding ceased and the hematocrit stabilized. However, when the WBC rose from 67,000 to 136,000 and daily temperature spikes to 102°F appeared, VAMP therapy was reinstituted. Within one day the gingiva again were bleeding and numerous fundal hemorrhages appeared. The PT was 19 sec, fibrinogen 264/dl, and platelets 32,000/ul. VAMP therapy was stopped. Death occurred several days later with a WBC of 263,000 and signs of intracerebral bleeding.

Autopsy showed acute promyelocytic leukemia involving bone marrow, lymph nodes, spleen, liver, kidneys, muscle, right thigh, gums, brain and subcutaneous tissues; fibrin thrombi in kidney and testes; bronchopneumonia.

Comment: This case is an example of DIC associated with acute promyelocytic leukemia. Two episodes of DIC were associated with institution of antileukemic therapy, one responding to heparin and EACA. Massive hematomata at venipuncture and injection sites heralded each episode.

CASE 22 (FIG. III-I)—E. COLI SEPTICEMIA: A 6-day-old white infant with Hirschsprung's disease entered with intestinal obstruction. At laparotomy the bowel contents were evacuated and twelve days later a definitive operation was performed. Postoperatively the hematocrit was 37% and the platelets were normal. One day later the WBC was 19,500 and platelets began falling. On the seventeenth day the abdomen became distended, the temperature was 99°F and the platelets had dropped to 53,000/ul. Blood cultures grew out *E. coli*. Penicillin was administered. During the ensuing day the platelets fell further. At laparotomy abscesses were found under the diaphragm and in the left gutter; cultures grew out *E. coli*, bacteroides, alpha-hemolytic streptococcus, and yeast. Gentamicin and chloramphenicol were administered.

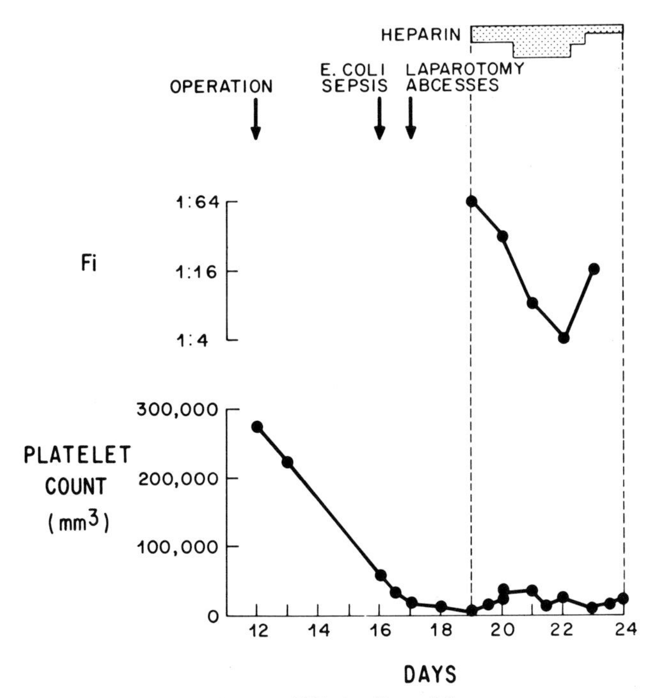

Figure III–1. Case 22

The hematocrit was 31%, WBC 5400, platelets 9000/ul, fibrinogen 100 mg/dl and Fi titer 1:64. There was no evidence of bleeding. Heparin (300 U every 4 hr) was begun. During the next two days the platelets rose slightly and the Fi fell. The dosage of heparin was increased to 450 U every 4 hrs. Although the cardiovascular status slowly improved, he remained grossly septic. Cultures from the tracheostomy, urine, and tube drainages continued to grow the spectrum of organisms noted previously. Because the Fi returned to a normal range, the dosage of heparin was lowered on the twenty-second day to 300 U and then 125 U every 4 hrs. Shortly thereafter the Fi rose to 1:16. No obvious change in the clinical course occurred, and sepsis continued. During the next day cyanosis appeared; the pH was 7.0 and a pneumothorax was discovered on the right side. Death occurred hours later.

Autopsy revealed Hirschsprung's disease; multiple peritoneal abscesses; acute bronchopneumonia; fibrin thrombi in adrenal gland and kidney; organizing thrombi in large arteries near the thyroid.

Comment: This case is an example of DIC associated with *E. coli* septicemia. Heparin therapy was associated with correction of severely abnormal coagulation tests and was well tolerated despite recent extensive surgery. When the dosage of heparin was decreased in the face of ongoing septicemia, coagulation tests again became abnormal.

CASE 35—TWO EPISODES OF DIC WITH SEVERE PROLONGED HYPOTENSION AND STAPHYLOCOCCAL ENDOCARDITIS: A 69 year old white female entered because of vomiting. Six weeks previously she had undergone an open commissurotomy for calcific mitral stenosis complicated postoperatively by jaundice. At discharge the hepatic function tests and PT were normal; the platelet count was 144,000/ul. Shortly thereafter she returned with hepatitis. Coagulation tests were normal. Methylprednisolone (60 mg daily) was started, and three weeks later liver function tests were again normal.

On the thirty-ninth day she vomited guaiac positive material, and one day later frank blood. For two hours no blood pressure could be obtained. Striking acral cyanosis, mottled livido reticularis, and the sudden onset of multiple 3–5 cm. hematomas at all venipuncture and cut-down sites appeared. There were no petechiae. The platelet count was 27,000/ul, fibrinogen 96 mg/dl, and PT 16 sec, Fi 1:32, ELT normal, and TT 24 sec. Hydrocortisone, transfusions, and heparin (4750 U, 2 doses) were started. The blood pressure returned, peripheral perfusion improved and wound bleeding stopped. By the next day the platelet count was 105,000/ul; fibrinogen 264 mg/dl and the Fi test, TT, PTT and PT were normal. She was placed on a bland diet, and the steroid dose was reduced. During the next days, the platelet count fell to 38,000/ul and thereafter remained at 38–70,000/ul; the other clotting tests remained normal.

On the forty-eighth day a fever of 101°F appeared, and she was confused. Cultures from the blood, intravenous canula tip and urine grew out *S. albus*. The hematocrit fell to 27% and petechiae developed on the palate and conjunctivae. The PT was 21 sec, platelets 20,000/ul, PTT 41 sec, fibrinogen 34 mg/dl, Fi 1:128, TT 37 sec, ELT 15 min. Heparin (4750 U every 4 hr) was started. Within a day after the petechiae were first noted, the urine output fell, and the blood pressure was 70 systolic, 40 diastolic. She became disoriented and had guaiac positive stools. Six units of whole blood and EACA (4 gm IV loading dose, then 1 gm hourly) were given. A new holosystolic murmur was heard, rectal bleeding progressed, and hematemesis began. The platelet count was 30,000/ul and fibrinogen 100 mg/dl. Death occurred on the fifty-sixth day.

Autopsy showed rheumatic heart disease with mitral stenosis; subacute *S. albus* endocarditis of mitral valve; multiple embolic infarcts in brain, spleen; fibrin thrombi in kidney; acute duodenal ulcer with gastrointestinal hemorrhage; minimal hepatitis.

Comment: This patient had two episodes of DIC. The first was associated with severe and prolonged hypotension secondary to a bleeding duodenal ulcer, and the second with *S. albus* endocarditis. In the first episode bleeding dramatically stopped and the clotting tests promptly returned to normal after heparin was given and the volume deficit corrected.

CASE 39—ACUTE MYELOGENOUS LEUKEMIA: A 41-year-old white female entered with abdominal pain, a temperature of 102°F, mild oozing from venipuncture sites, and purpura over the lower extremities. The hematocrit was 25%, WBC 124,000 with 98% myeloblasts, PT 12 sec, platelets 195,000/ul and fibrinogen 340 mg/dl. Six-thioguanine, cytosine arabinoside and transfusions were given and within four days the WBC was 24,000 with 90% blast cells, platelet count 59,000/ul, fibrinogen 230 mg/dl, Fi 1:32, and TT 25 sec. After an additional five days the hematocrit was 23%, WBC 2,000 with 10% blast cells, PT 14 sec, platelet count 21,000/ul, fibrinogen 96 mg/dl, TT, ELT and Fi normal.

Antileukemic therapy was stopped. Within four days the PT returned to 12 sec while the fibrinogen rose to 144 mg/dl. An aspirate of bone marrow was packed with blast cells and antileukemic therapy was reinstituted at half the previous dosage. No heparin therapy was given. Thirty days after admission, the WBC was 800 (without blast cells), platelet count 15,000/ul, PT 13 sec and fibrinogen 370 mg/dl. Death occurred one week later.

Autopsy showed acute myelogenous leukemia and fibrin thrombi in pancreas.

Comment: This case illustrates DIC triggered by chemotherapy for cancer.

Although acute progranulocytic leukemia is characteristically associated with DIC (161, 163, 167, 179), DIC also complicates other granulocytic leukemias, particularly myelomonocytic leukemia. In contrast, DIC is rarely associated with acute lymphoblastic leukemia, with epithelial tumors other than prostate (51), or as a complication of massive surgery or extracorporeal circulation.

Conditions we have not encountered, but which have a high incidence of DIC are giant hemangiomas (12, 184), heat stroke, accidental hypothermia, snake bite (111), fat embolism (180), viral hemorrhagic fevers (118), extensive burns, and aortic aneurysms. Disease settings that will probably be seen more frequently with DIC are the syndrome of splenectomy and septicemic DIC (11), and rejection of transplanted organs (particularly kidney) with either local (intraorgan) (21, 27) or generalized (28, 190) DIC.

Thrombotic thrombocytopenic purpura (TTP), like DIC, is a syndrome (206) caused by diverse etiologies. Although many cases are not associated with DIC, a considerable overlap definitely exists (152). DIC can masquerade as the syndrome of TTP (176) (see history of Case 28, Chap. X). Therefore, if coagulation tests indicate the presence of DIC in a suspected case of TTP, occult underlying diseases should be considered.

Similarly, if DIC or fibrinolysis appear to be "primary" or "idiopathic," a vigorous search for an underlying disease is indicated. Frequently neoplasia is found if the process is chronic (135), or infection if the process is acute. If bacterial or viral septicemia appear unlikely in cases of acute DIC without an obvious etiology, fungal invasion of blood vessels should be considered (159, 176).

In identifying the various processes that are temporally related to the episode of DIC, it is helpful to identify not only the "primary" underlying disease, but also other events which may have "precipitated" or "predisposed" the patient to the DIC. Hypotension (38, 39), hypoxia, acidosis (18), liver damage (134, 166, 208), and splenectomy (11) are often found. Cancer chemotherapy frequently appears to trigger DIC (102), presumably by liberating massive amounts of tissue thromboplastin from leukemic cells or other procoagulants during tumor lysis. Catheterization of vessels for obtaining central venous pressure, arterial pressure, or blood gases is now commonplace in the treatment of the critically ill patient. The thrombosis of major vessels that sometimes occurs at these sites in patients with DIC can have catastrophic clinical consequences. Catheterization should be highly suspect as a factor aggravating or unmasking DIC, and such manipulation should be avoided whenever possible in patients suspected of having DIC.

Summary

DIC is a symptom of an underlying disease and not a disease in itself. Several clinical states, especially septicemia, hypotension, and certain malignancies, should be held highly suspect of developing DIC. When the etiology of DIC is obscure, search should be made for an occult disease. Frequently, multiple etiologies for DIC are present in the individual patient.

CHAPTER IV

CLINICAL FEATURES

MODE OF PRESENTATION

DIC CAN BE SUSPECTED ON clinical grounds with a high degree of accuracy. The mode of presentation of DIC in our patients was usually an acute bleeding or purpuric diathesis (Table IV-I) associated with sepsis, hypotension or neoplasia. Chronic bleeding diatheses and thrombotic presentations without bleeding are less common. Occasionally, abnormal coagulation tests alone herald the onset of DIC; unpredictable courses follow ranging from the appearance of massive bleeding to resolution of the coagulation abnormalities without bleeding. With an increased awareness that DIC occurs in certain clinical situations, more episodes will be detected early by coagulation tests. The therapeutic approach to such patients is discussed in Chapter XI.

TIME COURSE OF HEMORRHAGIC MANIFESTATIONS

The duration of bleeding, acral cyanosis, or thrombosis from the onset of DIC until it is clinically recognized varies from minutes to weeks. In most cases (85%) the duration is less than two days. The acute onset of DIC is best explained by the acute nature of the most frequent underlying etiologies, e.g. septicemia, hypotension (see history of Case 19), or destruction of neoplastic tissues by chemotherapy. Chronic bleeding lasting three or more weeks is less common (15%). When abnormal coagulation values are the initial sign of DIC, bleeding or other manifestations usually develop within the ensuing week.

CASE 19—DISSECTING AORTIC ANEURYSM: A 75 year old black woman with a known thoracic aortic aneurysm entered with inter-

TABLE IV-I

CARDINAL MANIFESTATIONS OF DIC

Manifestations	Presenting sign (54 episodes) %		Eventual Manifestations (54 episodes) %	
Bleeding	78		87	
Single site (excluding purpura)		6		6
Purpura or petechiae only		20		2
Multiple sites[1]		52		79
Acral cyanosis	7		14	
Thrombosis (clinically evident)	2		22	
Abnormal lab value only	13		8	
	100%			

[1] All purpura and petechiae counted as one site.

scapular back pain. The blood pressure was 170 systolic, 110 diastolic and a loud systolic, ejection murmur was audible at the cardiac apex. The hematocrit was 34%, WBC 6400, PT 15 sec, and platelets 310,000/ul. Several hours after admission, she suffered a cardiac arrest, was promptly resuscitated, and one hour later was alert. Suddenly bleeding appeared at all venipuncture sites and a large hematoma developed at a cutdown site. The hematocrit was 27%, PT 15 sec, platelets 55,000/ul, fibrinogen 110 mg/dl, and TT and ELT normal. No heparin was given. During the next two days the platelets rose to 129,000/ul, fibrinogen to 198 mg/dl, but the PT remained elevated at 16 sec. One week later she underwent thoracotomy for an iatrogenic cardiac tamponade, peritoneal dialysis for acute tubular necrosis, and died without having recurrent DIC.

Autopsy showed an organizing dissecting aneurysm of thoracic and abdominal aorta. Fibrin thrombi were found only in the skin.

Comment: This case is an example of DIC occurring immediately after cardiac arrest, shock and hypotension. With correction of the precipitating event the DIC clinically abated.

EVALUATION, LOCATION AND EVOLUTION OF HEMORRHAGIC-THROMBOTIC MANIFESTATIONS

The recognition that an acquired hemorrhagic diathesis exists is often delayed in three common situations. First, the critically ill patient often has multiple catheters, venipuncture sites and surgical wounds. Ooozing of blood can occur at these sites but the presence of a bleeding diathesis goes unrecognized because the hemorrhage is attributed to wounds and catheters alone. Similarly, thrombosis of vessels is often attributed solely to the mechanical effects of catheters. Secondly, when a patient suffers a major hemorrhage from a local site (e.g., gastrointestinal tract ulcer), other sites of concomitant bleeding (purpura, hematomas) are overlooked because they lack the drama of the local site hemorrhage. Such a combination of massive hematemesis and venipuncture site bleeding occurred in several of our patients. A third situation that can be misleading is the occurrence of acral cyanosis, which can be mistakenly attributed to hypoxemia or hypotension alone. The combination of septicemia and acral cyanosis is increasingly recognized as a sign of DIC. When hypoxemia has been corrected, large vessel pulses are intact, and blood pressure is adequate, the persistence of acral cyanosis or development of a gangrenous digit is highly suggestive of DIC (also see "Dermatologic Manifestations" in Chap. IV).

The bleeding associated with DIC is usually clinically obvious since the skin is involved in the vast majority (84%) of the bleeding episodes. Although the skin findings usually herald the onset of DIC, dramatic bleeding may occur at other sites, especially as massive hematemesis or hemoptysis (*see* history of Case 35 in Chap. III, and Case 24 in Chap. IV). Other common sites of bleeding include the lower gastrointestinal tract, genitourinary tract, and mucosal surfaces throughout the body (Table IV-II). The finding of multisite bleeding is of great diagnostic importance since patients with DIC usually bleed from multiple sites. In order to detect these sites one must specifically examine the skin, mucous membranes, wounds, venipuncture and intravenous administration sites, vagina, urine, tracheal aspirates and stool for blood.

Pulmonary and central nervous system bleeding play a large role in the mortality attributable to DIC (*see* Chap. IX and Chap. X). Evaluation of these potential sites is crucial. Unexplained infiltrates on chest X-ray, blood in the sputum or tracheal aspirates, and rales in the absence of congestive heart failure or infection may suggest pulmonary hemorrhage. Careful neurologic and funduscopic examination, together with

TABLE IV-II

BLEEDING SITES DURING DIC

	Episodes (54)		
	No.		Frequency (%)
Purpura - petechiae	34		63
Gastrointestinal - total	27		50
Upper GI		13	
Lower GI		7	
Upper + Lower		7	
Wound	25		46
Hematuria	17		32
Hematomas	14		26
Hemoptysis - Pulmonary	13		24
Mucosal	11		20
Vaginal	6		10
Epistaxis	5		9
Central Nervous System	4		7
Fundus of Eye	4		7
Pleural Cavity	3		6
Pericardial	1		2
Hemarthrosis	1		2

examination of the cerebrospinal fluid, if warranted by neurologic findings, are mandatory to detect CNS bleeding. Pericardial hemorrhage and airway obstruction from hematomas are rarely encountered, but should be considered if signs of such develop in patients with DIC.

Thrombosis of major blood vessels is rarely the presenting sign of DIC, but appears during the course of DIC in over a fifth of the patients (Table IV-III, *see also* "Pathology of major blood vessels" in Chap. X). Usually the arterial and venous thromboses occur at the sites of intravascular cannulae (*see* histories of Cases 38 and 43). The histories of two patients (Cases 28, 45) with thrombosis associated with aspergillus septicemia are presented in Chapter X.

CASE 38—MAJOR VESSEL THROMBOSIS AND PULMONARY EMBOLISM ASSOCIATED WITH VENOUS CATHETER: A 53-year-old white man entered with third degree burns covering 10% of the body. On admission the hematocrit was 44%, WBC 23,300, PT normal, platelets 260,000/ul, fibrinogen 200 mg/dl, SGOT 1400 U, LDH 800 U, and CPK 565 U. A central venous pressure catheter was radiographically in the superior vena cava. An electrocardiogram revealed an acute myocardial infarct, and a chest X-ray showed pulmonary edema. He was intubated and given methylpredniso-lone, cephalothin, and silver nitrate soaks. During the next two

TABLE IV-III

MAJOR VESSEL THROMBOSES ASSOCIATED WITH DIC

	Patients (45)		
	No.	Frequency %	Case #
Venous thrombosis[1]	6	13	8,22,23,36,38,43
Arterial thrombosis[2]	7	16	8,15,28,32,33,43,45
Pulmonary emboli[3]	5	11	1,8B,33,36,38

[1] All were associated with central venous pressure catheter; 4 were clinically evident, and 2 were associated with the large eschars of purpura fulminans.

[2] Two were associated with aspergillus in vessels, two with arterial cannulae, and one each with renal aneurysm, arterial puncture, and EACA therapy. Three of these patients (8,33,43) developed acral gangrene.

[3] Three of the pulmonary emboli were associated with thrombi at the tips of central venous pressure catheters (33,36,38).

days he developed acidosis, hypotension and low urine output. On the third day chest pain occurred and an acute pulmonary embolus was suspected clinically. Cultures of sputum and urine grew *E. coli* and *Ps. aeruginosa*, respectively and chloramphenicol was begun. The PT was 18 sec, platelets 110,000/ul, and fibrinogen 640 mg/dl.

The cardiac status slowly deteriorated and on the seventh day cardiac arrest occurred. Resuscitation was successful. Twelve hours later petechiae and ecchymoses appeared on the legs near intramuscular injection sites and a large hematoma appeared at an intravenous cannula site. The PT was 25 sec, platelets 65,000/ul, fibrinogen 200 mg/dl, TT 23 sec, PTT and ELT normal, and Fi titer 1:32. One day later green pustules appeared on the left arm, chest X-ray disclosed bilateral patchy infiltrates, and death occurred.

Autopsy showed an acute myocardial infarct and third degree burns of the skin, fibrin thrombi in renal glomerular and testicular capillaries, extensive thrombus about the central venous pressure catheter in the superior vena cava, and pulmonary emboli.

Comment: Thrombosis occurred about a central venous pressure catheter during DIC and pulmonary embolism followed. In addition, the fibrinogen level of 200 mg/dl that was recorded during the episode of DIC was within normal limits, but represented for this patient a state of "relative hypofibrinogenemia" since three days earlier the level had been 640 mg/dl.

CASE 43 (FIG. IV-I)—ARTERIAL THROMBOSIS ASSOCIATED WITH A VESSEL CATHETER: A 51 year-old white woman entered with a massive right lower lobe *S. aureus* pneumonia. The hematocrit was 37%, WBC 4100, PT 13 sec, platelets 123,000/ul, and fibrinogen 400 mg/dl. Kanamycin, oxacillin and assisted ventilation were

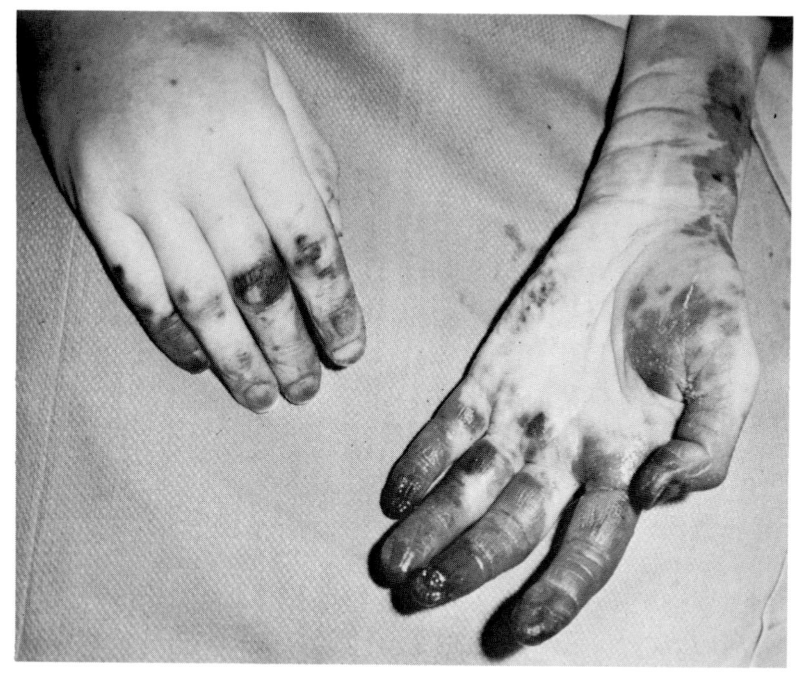

Figure IV–1. Acral cyanosis, hemorrhagic bullae and gangrene in DIC. The irregular borders (so called "geographic configuration") are sharply demarcated from the uninvolved skin. Case 43. (Robboy, Mihm, Colman, and Minna: *Br J Dermatol*, *88*:221, 1973).

begun. A left radial artery catheter (for monitoring blood gases) and a central venous pressure catheter in the superior vena cava were placed. On the third day the blood pressure dropped to 90 systolic, 60 diastolic and metaraminol was given. Despite the administration of 100% oxygen, the pO_2 remained below 40 mm mercury. X-rays of the chest showed extensive bilateral pneumonia. On the fourth day, the blood pressure fell to 60 systolic and an electrocardiogram revealed subendocardial ischemia. The platelets were 186,000/ul.

On the seventh day respirations became labored and a massive pneumothorax was found. The fingertips of the left hand were markedly cyanotic, despite palpable radial artery pulses. Metaraminol and epinephrine were given, and slight improvement was noted. During the next day the fingers of both hands (but especially the left) and then the toes of the right foot became ecchymotic and gangrenous. No other bleeding was observed. The PT was 24 sec, PTT > 2 min, platelets 90,500/ul, fibrinogen 140 mg/dl and Fi titer 1:16. Heparin (9000 U every 4 hr) and chloramphenicol were administered. Within one day, the skin lesions stabilized and some showed slight improvement, despite increasing respiratory distress. On the ninth day the PT was 19 sec and platelets 185,000/ul. On the twelfth day heparin was stopped. The distal portions of the digits of the left hand began undergoing liquefication necrosis (Fig. IV-I). Death occurred on the next day.

Autopsy showed a massive *S. aureus* bronchopneumonia; fibrin thrombi in renal glomerular capillaries and in capillaries, venules and veins of both hands and right foot; organizing thromboses of left radial artery (about cannula); organizing thrombus about right subclavian vein (about catheter); and organizing thrombus in left popliteal vein.

Comment: This case is an example of DIC presenting as acral cyanosis upon a background of massive *S. aureus* bronchopneumonia and coronary artery atherosclerosis. Large arteries or veins into which cannulas or catheters had been inserted were thrombosed.

SEVERITY OF BLEEDING

Bleeding occurs in most patients with DIC (87%) (Table IV-IV). Quantitative evaluation of severity of bleeding is important in determining prognosis and in judging response to therapy. One-third of our patients demonstrated severe bleeding; none survived to leave the hospital. In contrast, about half of the patients with no, mild or moderate bleeding left the hospital (Table I-II). Exsanguinating hemorrhage is usually obvious, but lesser degrees of hemorrhage are often underestimated. Patients may appear to have only mild bleeding by physical examination, but after the fall in hematocrit,

TABLE IV-IV

SEVERITY OF BLEEDING MANIFESTATIONS

Combined Score[1] of bleeding severity	Episodes (54)	
	No.	Frequency (%)
None	7	13
Mild	14	26
Moderate	16	30
Severe	17	31

[1] None, no bleeding; mild, oozing of blood; moderate, bleeding requiring transfusion, or confluent purpura with fall in hematocrit of > 10%; severe, exsanguinating hemorrhage clinically or brisk bleeding from ≥ 3 sites with fall in HCT by > 10%, or transfusion requirement of 10 units of blood and/or plasma per episode. The presence of petechiae-purpura was scored as only one bleeding site despite the number of lesions.

transfusion requirement and the number of bleeding sites are tabulated, a substantial blood loss can be recognized. In our experience, a patient should be considered as having severe bleeding with DIC (and thus an ominous prognosis) if there is bleeding from three or more sites and fall in hematocrit by greater than 10%, or transfusion requirement of 10 units of blood and/or plasma per episode.

SIGNS AND SYMPTOMS

Most patients with DIC are critically ill with multiple associated underlying disease states, all of which also have clinical signs and symptoms. Table IV-V lists signs, symptoms, or laboratory data that were evaluated in each patient. In nearly all instances, a coexisting pathologic situation other than DIC is a sufficient explanation for the manifestations (*see also* "Organ dysfunction" (Chap. IX).

The syndrome of acute multiorgan dysfunction (oliguria, dyspnea, confusion, coma, convulsions, abdominal pain, back pain and diarrhea) which McKay (116) has described has not been encountered. Fever is found frequently (58%) but is nearly always associated with documented sepsis. Hypotension also occurs frequently (50%) but can usually be ascribed to on-going septicemia, cardiogenic shock, hemorrhage, or hypovolemia (Table IV-VI). Since the hypotension associated with DIC is reversible in many instances (56% of our patients), the underlying causes of hypotension should be treated vigorously.

Hypoxemia, dyspnea, congestive heart failure,oliguria, and azotemia occur commonly, but in most patients were due to atherosclerotic coronary heart disease, organ sepsis, or hypovolemia. Obviously these signs of serious disease have diagnostic and therapeutic implications in the DIC patient. As will be discussed in Chapter IX, pulmonary and central nervous system hemorrhage lead to the only recognizable organ dysfunction that can be consistently attributed to DIC.

DERMATOLOGIC MANIFESTATIONS

Examination of the skin can be of great diagnostic value in patients with DIC. The eight lesions that are encountered

TABLE IV-V
CLINICAL SYMPTOMS AND SIGNS IN DIC (EXCLUDING BLEEDING)

	Occurrence/Episode		Frequency (%)
Fever (all cases)	32/54	"	58
Without Sepsis	4/32	"	12
Hypotension	27/54	"	50
Acidosis (pH < 7.3)	9/18	"	50
Cardiopulmonary			
Hypoxemia (pO_2 < 80 mm Hg with > 40% inspired O_2)	9/15	"	60
Dyspnea	17/50	"	33
Pulmonary Congestion	17/54	"	33
Arrhythmia (EKG)	10/44	"	23
Assisted Ventilation	13/45	Patients	28
Elevated Venous Pressure	12/45	"	26
Cardiogenic shock syndrome	10/45	"	22
Cardiomegaly	9/45	"	20
Edema	11/54	Episodes	19
Block (EKG)	6/44	"	17
Ischemia (EKG)	6/44	"	17
Pleural effusion	6/45	"	16
Chest pain	4/45	"	9
Hepatic			
Jaundice	12/45	Patients	26
Hepatomegaly	10/45	"	22
Splenomegaly	10/45	"	22
Hepatic coma	3/45	"	6
Gastrointestinal			
Vomiting	12/54	Episodes	21
Abdominal pain	8/48	"	15
Acute abdominal signs	8/51	"	14
Diarrhea	0/54	"	0
Renal			
Proteinuria	22/45	"	51
Azotemia	18/50	"	38
Oliguria	16/51	"	31
Casts	2/45	"	5
Neurologic			
Coma	19/54	"	35
Focal neurologic	15/54	"	29
Confusion - delirium	9/54	"	15
Stroke Syndrome	5/54	"	9
Seizures	2/54	"	4
Dermatologic			
Palpable purpura	7/45	Patients	16
Necrotic - gangrenous	7/45	"	16
Hemorrhagic bullae	4/45	"	9
Arthralgia - myalgia	9/44	Episodes	21
Back pain	6/40	"	13

regularly are petechiae, purpura, palpable purpura, hemorrhagic bullae, acral cyanosis, gangrene, wound and venipuncture bleeding, and subcutaneous hematomas (173) (Table IV-VII). With the exception of petechiae and purpura, the acquired presence of any of the other skin lesions is highly suggestive of DIC. Skin biopsy and coagulation tests will lead to the appropriate diagnosis.

TABLE IV-VI
ETIOLOGY OF HYPOTENSION ASSOCIATED WITH DIC

Condition associated with hypotension	Number of patients	Number of patients with reversible hypotension
Septicemic	11	8
Cardiogenic	8	3
Hemorrhagic	5	3
Miscellaneous		
massive pneumothorax	1	1
Unexplained		
purpura fulminans	1	0
stroke syndrome	1	0
	27	15

Petechiae are minute, sometimes pinpoint-sized, flat lesions caused by hemorrhage into the skin, while purpura are the larger skin hemorrhages. Raised or "palpable" petechiae and purpura are of particular importance since biopsy of them often disclose fibrin thrombi. Hemorrhagic bullae are blisters filled with blood. Purpura fulminans is extensive confluent purpura of explosive onset that is frequently associated with hemorrhagic bullous formation and focal gangrene.

Acral cyanosis refers to gun-metal gray to purplish discolorations of the digits and occasionally, ears or nose that do not blanch with pressure. In these cases the large arterial pulses of the involved extremities are usually normal. These lesions have irregular borders that are often sharply demarked

TABLE IV-VII
CUTANEOUS MANIFESTATIONS OF DIC[1]

	Episodes (54)	
	Number	Frequency (%)
Any skin lesions related to DIC	36	67
Purpura/petechiae	34	63
Wound/venipuncture bleeding	16	30
Palpable purpura	10	18
Subcutaneous hematoma	10	18
Acral cyanosis	9	17
Hemorrhagic bullae	7	13
Gangrene	6	11
Initial symptoms of DIC related to skin	17	32

[1] Of the 36 patients with cutaneous manifestations, 6 had meningococcemia, 11 other forms of septicemia, 7 acute granulocytic leukemia, 5 epithelial carcinomas, 2 purpura fulminans, and 5 miscellaneous diseases.

from the uninvolved skin (so called "geographic distribution"). Dissecting hematomas are extensive subcutaneous accumulations of blood that appeared rapidly as progressive, painful tumefactions.

Petechiae and/or purpura are the most common skin lesions found in DIC, occurring in 63 percent of all episodes of DIC and 94 percent of the episodes in which the skin is involved. Of importance, the rapid appearance of petechiae/purpura is the immediate cause prompting many patients to seek medical advice. Usually the petechiae and purpura remain confined to the extremities, although sometimes they spread in a centripetal fashion or are generalized. On occasion the purpura progress to hemorrhagic bullae and in rare instances into purpura fulminans. In meningococcemia and purpura fulminans, the petechiae and purpura are usually palpable (see histories of Cases 6, 26, and 31 below).

Acral cyanosis is a striking lesion that occurs in 17 percent of the episodes of DIC, and is most frequently associated with concomitant septicemia and hypotension (Tables IV-VII, V-II). Not uncommonly acral cyanosis can evolve into gangrene of the acral regions, including the nose. The presence of either in-dwelling arterial or venous catheters in an involved extremity is associated with more extensive acral cyanosis and gangrenous complications. Not infrequently patients with acral cyanosis who improve have gangrenous digital tips that self-amputate or eventually require surgical amputation (Fig. IV-I). Since patients can survive such episodes, they should be vigorously treated for septicemia, hypotension, and DIC.

CASE 6—PURPURA FULMINANS: A 74 year-old man entered with extensive confluent purpura. Six weeks prior to admission sulfisoxazole therapy was begun and continued for three weeks because of melena related to suspected diverticulitis. Five days before admission, facial swelling with pruritus and fever appeared, for which diphenylhydramine was prescribed. Three days later scrotal swelling appeared followed by multiple purpura and subcutaneous hemorrhages involving the flanks, scrotum, groin and thighs

On admission the confluent palpable purpura were maximally 25 cm in diameter, bullous with dark blue centers and irregular, poorly defined edges. The vital signs and rest of physical examination were normal. The hematocrit was 28%; the peripheral smear showed numerous oval and bizarre red cells. The WBC was 23,500 with 85% neutrophils, PT 27 sec, platelets 52,000/ul, fibrinogen 86 mg/dl, PTT 64 sec, and Factor VIII 15%. Skin biopsy showed multiple fibrin thrombi in the capillaries and venules of the papillary and reticular dermis, extensive extravasation of erythrocytes, and subepidermal bullae.

Heparin (6000 U every 4 hr), fresh whole blood (2 units), fibrinogen (4 gm), and vitamin K_1 were administered. On the third day the skin sloughed in the areas of ecchymoses and left dark blue-black scars. The temperature rose to 101 – 102°F and remained so until death. The PT fell to 16 sec, the platelet count rose to 290,000/ul and the fibrinogen to 290 mg/dl. On the fourth day cultures of the throat and skin grew out abundant beta hemolytic streptococci group B. The ASLO titer was < 100 Todd units. Components C1 and C4 of complement were markedly decreased; C2, C3 and C8 were only mildly decreased. Penicillin was started and the heparin was increased (6250 U every 4 hr). The old areas of ecchymosis which involved 40% of the total body surface became gangrenous and sloughed (Fig. X-17).

On the sixth day eight new skin lesions appeared. The hematocrit was 26%, PT 17 sec, platelets 160,000/ul, fibrinogen 140 mg/dl, and Fi titer 1:80. The heparin was increased to 10,000 U every 4 hours, and dextran was administered along with fresh whole blood. One day later he became hypotensive, started oozing blood from his multiple skin lesions, vomited and died.

Autopsy revealed purpura fulminans with fibrin thrombi in skin, testes, colon, pericardium, adventitia of aorta, adrenal, lung, and spleen; portal fibrosis of liver.

Comment: This patient had classic "purpura fulminans." The history was suggestive of an allergic reaction and subsequently beta streptococcal infection was documented. The bleeding that occurred into the skin and subcutaneous tissue was massive and the necrotic lesions are essentially similar to massive third degree burns. The initial episode of DIC responded quickly to heparin and blood products administration. When new skin lesions appeared on the sixth day, all coagulation tests deteriorated, despite heparin therapy. This suggests that the dosage of heparin had become inadequate, a phenomenon observed in other cases with recurrent DIC (*see* history of Case 13 in Chap. VI).

CASE 26—MENINGOCOCCAL MENINGITIS AND SKIN LESIONS OF DIC: A 39-year-old woman was admitted because of purpura. Six days previously myalgia, arthralgia and rhinitis had appeared, followed by a 102°F fever. On the morning of admission multiple purpura appeared on the palms of the hands and rapidly spread. At admission the blood pressure was 50 systolic, 10 diastolic.

Petechiae and purpura were diffuse, affecting even the conjunctiva. The extremities were most severely involved while the trunk was relatively spared. Various types of purpuric lesions were seen. Some were flat, others palpable; some had clear and others necrotic centers. The extremities, especially the fingers, feet and nose, displayed 3–4 cm patches of cyanosis characterized by a central gun-metal gray color and erythematous, purplish borders. The lesions were neither pruritic nor painful and did not blanch. The radial and dorsalis pedis artery pulses were intact. Pneumonia and 50 ml of blood in the vagina were also present. Cultures of spinal fluid grew *Neisseria meningitidis*.

Therapy with both penicillin and heparin (5000 U every 4 hr) was begun. During the first days new purpura erupted over acral regions, leading to confluent purpura of the extremities that evolved into hemorrhagic bullae. Because the vaginal bleeding persisted the uterus was curetted, but only secretory endometrium was found. By the second day she was dramatically improved. The numerous purpura and other skin lesions began to fade. The hematocrit, which had fallen from an initial value of 39 to 23%, rose to 30%. The PT fell from 19 sec to normal and the fibrinogen rose from 130 to 480 mg/dl. The platelet count was unchanged at 36,000/ul, not rising to normal for an additional 5 days.

During the ensuing week the purpura that had most recently appeared, disappeared. However, purpura and hemorrhagic bullae in acral regions became extremely tender and gangrenous. On the eighth day heparin therapy was discontinued. By the end of the second week several acral lesions showed deep necrosis and the tips of all but one toe had dry gangrene. She was discharged after five weeks; two months later the tips of the toes were surgically amputated.

Comment: This case illustrates the diagnostic importance of the various skin lesions in DIC, and their mode of appearance, evolution and regression.

CASE 31 (FIG. IV-2)—ACRAL CYANOSIS, PNEUMOCOCCAL SEPTICEMIA, AND SPLENECTOMY: A 32 year-old white woman entered with shaking chills of one day's duration. Twelve years previously, splenectomy was performed because of abdominal trauma. Upon admission to another hospital, the blood pressure was 80 systolic, 60 diastolic, the hands and feet were cyanotic, petechiae dotted the nose and cheeks, and WBC was 25,000. Blood cultures grew *Pneumococcus pneumoniae*. Despite penicillin, cephalothin, and methylprednisolone therapy, the feet remained cyanotic and painful.

Upon admission to this hospital one day later the blood pressure was normal. Palpable 2–3 mm purpura were present on the nose and cheeks. The nasal mucosa was focally necrotic and bleeding. There was marked cyanosis of the lips, ears, tip of nose and hands.

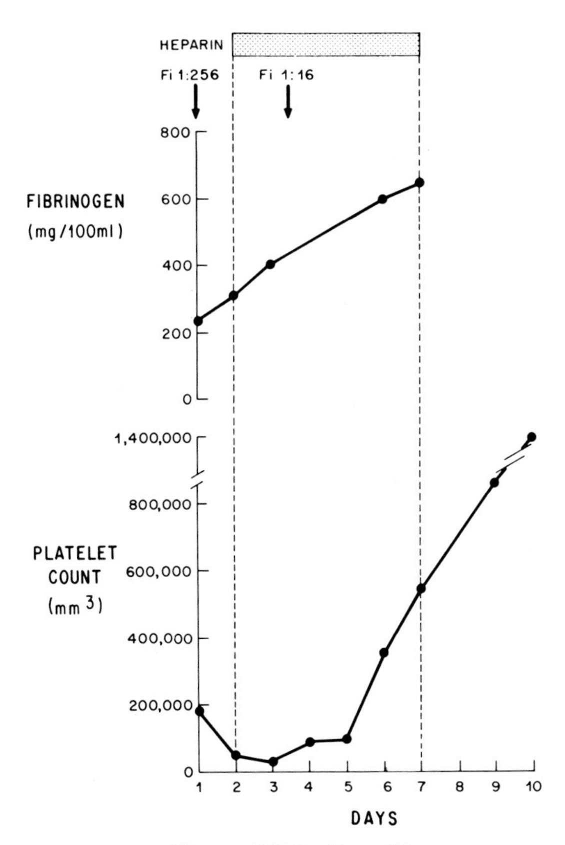

Figure IV–2. Case 31

The legs were cool below the knees, confluently purpuric below the calves and anesthetic below the ankles. The second, third and fourth toes of both feet were dark blue-black and had the appearance of impending gangrene.

There were numerous splinter hemorrhages under the fingernails and perifollicular hemorrhages on the proximal extremities. The cyanotic acral areas were markedly tender to deep palpation; upon release of pressure, capillary filling did not occur. The arterial pulses, including the dorsalis pedis, were strong. Biopsy of cheek and leg skin revealed fibrin thrombi in numerous dermal capillaries and venules, focal eosinophilic smudginess of several of the vessel walls, minimal extravasation of erythrocytes and rare perivascular neutrophils and lymphocytes. One of the specimens showed also subepidermal bullae which lacked signs of regeneration.

The hematocrit was 42% and the WBC 73,000 with 19% neutrophils and 77% band forms. The peripheral blood smear contained a few Howell-Jolly bodies, and rare schistocytes. The spinal fluid contained 25 red cells and 17 neutrophils. The SGOT was 131 U and the CPK 44 U. The platelet count was 191,000/ul, Fi titer 1:256, PT, PTT, ELT and TT normal, pO_2 75 mmHg and pH 7.34. After dextran, penicillin and chloramphenicol were given, the legs and feet became less painful and sensation returned. On the second day, the temperature rose to 101°F. Bleeding necrotic lesions appeared on the nasal septum and inferior turbinates. The mottled cyanosis of the feet persisted and the tips of several toes became black. The platelet count fell to 51,000/ul. Oxacillin and chloramphenicol were discontinued and heparin (4750 U every 4 hr) was given.

During the next three days, each of the skin lesions disappeared except for those of the gangrenous toes. Four days later, when the heparin was discontinued, the platelet count was 595,000/ul, fibrinogen 713 mg/dl, and CPK 35 U. On the twelfth day the penicillin was discontinued; the platelet count was 1,363,000/ul. Three months later, the tips of the gangrenous toes were amputated.

Comment: This case is an example of the syndrome of DIC, splenectomy and pneumococcal septicemia. It illustrates also the characteristic skin findings in DIC including acral cyanosis.

Frequently patients are already in the hospital when the event that triggers DIC occurs, e.g., chemotherapy for tumor, (*see* history of Case 27, Chap. IX). Usually abnormal coagulation values are already known when the bleeding from wounds or venipuncture sites begins. In one striking case the patient entered the hospital for a presumed myocardial infarct and was given an intramuscular injection wereupon bleeding began at this site and then developed into massive dissecting subcutaneous hematomas (*see* history of Case 24 below). Occasionally the skin manifestations are the first sign of DIC (see history of Case 36 below).

CASE 24 (TABLE IV-VIII)—PROSTATIC CARCINOMA WITH DISSECTING SUBCUTANEOUS HEMORRHAGE, SYSTEMIC FIBRINOLYSIS, AND PULMONARY HEMORRHAGE: A 68-year-old man entered with the acute onset of hemoptysis and right-sided chest pain. Three years previously, radical prostatectomy was performed for poorly differentiated adenocarcinoma which involved all lobes and had penetrated the capsule. The acid phosphatase was 0.24 U and the alkaline phosphatase 0.44 U. No postoperative therapy was given.

On admission Demerol® was given and within minutes, a massive hematoma appeared at the intramuscular injection site. No other sites of bleeding were evident. Examination revealed a rock hard

TABLE IV-VIII
CASE 24

	PT (sec)	Platelet count (per ul)	Fibrin-ogen (mg/dl)	ELT (min)	Fi
Admission	47	147,000		Immed	> 1:128
+ 9 hr	27	120,000	240	>120	
+ 18 hr	15	160,000	240		
+ 24 hr	12	146,000		>120	1:128
+ 2 day	12	117,000	370	>120	1:128
+ 3 day	12	101,000	490	>120	1:64
+ 5 day	12	79,000	550		
+ 6 day	12	155,000	360	>120	1:16
+ 7 day	12	215,000			1:8
+ 10 day		435,000		>120	

prostate, decreased breath sounds and rales in the right base. The respiratory rate was 24. A chest X-ray showed scattered opacifications throughout the lung, consistent with hemorrhage. The hematocrit was 41%, and the tests of coagulation abnormal (Table IV-VIII). Heparin (12,500 U) was given and then reduced in dosage (9000 U every 4 hr). Two hours later, the hematoma enlarged and new hematomas developed at venipuncture sites. The hematocrit fell to 32% and eight units of blood and plasma were administered. The ELT returned to normal.

On the second day conjugated estrogens and stilbestrol were given. During the next morning, the hematomas enlarged dissecting through the back and flank. On the fourth day a new dissecting hematoma appeared but all coagulation tests, except the platelet count, were improved. The heparin was continued. On the fifth day, hemoptysis recurred, the respiratory rate rose to 32, extensive rales developed bilaterally and serial X-rays showed progressive bilateral intra-alveolar infiltration. There were no other signs suggesting cardiac failure. The platelet count fell to 79,000/ul.

On the seventh day, the bleeding stopped, the hematocrit stabilized at 27% and the coagulation tests were normal, except for the platelet count. The heparin was decreased to 6000 U every 4 hr, and stopped after ten days of therapy. The BUN and creatinine which had risen to 142 and 5.9 mg/dl, respectively, fell to normal levels. The chest X-ray became normal and there were no further pulmonary symptoms. The patient was discharged after three weeks, was given 5000 R to the prostatic bed, and is presently asymptomatic.

Comment: This case illustrates dissecting subcutaneous hemorrhages, an unusual dermatologic manifestation of DIC, and systemic fibrinolysis and the pulmonary hemorrhage syndrome. Vigorous heparin therapy must sometimes be prolonged to control DIC.

CASE 36—GRAM NEGATIVE SEPTICEMIA, ACRAL GANGRENE AND PULMONARY EMBOLI: An 81-year-old man was admitted several times during the previous ten years for genitourinary tract septicemia, myocardial infarcts, and congestive heart failure. Two days before admission and 5 minutes after cystostomy tube irrigation, he experienced rigors, and chest pain.

On admission the temperature was 101°F. There was striking acral cyanosis and impending gangrene of the left fifth toe but no bleeding. The hematocrit was 30%, WBC 12,200 and rare helmet cells were observed. The PT and PTT were normal, platelets 226,000/ul, and fibrinogen 580 mg/dl. Chloramphenicol and plasma were given. Two hours later he had severe rigors, striking diffuse mottled cyanosis, and the blood pressure fell from 100 to 70 systolic and 60 diastolic. The acral cyanosis became worse and the toes were blue-black. Isoproterenol was administered and the blood pressure rose to 110 systolic, 70 diastolic, and the peripheral perfusion greatly improved; the tips of the toes remained blue. The platelets (188,000/ul) and fibrinogen (420 mg/dl) had fallen slightly.

On the third day generalized seizures occurred, followed by pulmonary edema, poor peripheral perfusion and severe metabolic acidosis (pH 7.13). The central venous pressure and other intravenous lines became thrombosed and symptoms of pulmonary emboli developed. Heparin (4750 U every 4 hr) was started. During the ensuing eight hours the peripheral perfusion improved dramatically and the toes became normal in color. Over the next three days the fibrinogen rose to 980 mg/dl and the heparin was stopped.

On the fourteenth day fever, rigors, hypotension (blood pressure 60 systolic, 10 diastolic) and acral cyanosis reappeared. The PT rose to 18 sec, the fibrinogen fell to 340 mg/dl, platelets fell to 144,000/ul, and the Fi titer was 1:32. Cultures of the blood and sputum grew klebsiella. Colistin, cephalothin, six units of plasma, and heparin (6000 U every 4 hr) were begun. The blood pressure rose, the peripheral perfusion returned, and over a five-day period the PT became normal, the platelets rose to 600,000/ul and the fibrinogen to 620 mg/dl. The cephalothin was stopped and he was discharged after five weeks. Three months later, a toe underwent autoamputation.

Comment: This patient illustrates the importance of acral cyanosis and its sequela, acral gangrene, as indicators of DIC. During the first episode of septicemia, DIC was absent by the usual coagulation criteria. Yet, the appearance of acral cyanosis, thrombosis around the CVP catheter, and the dramatic response of the fibrinogen after initiation of heparin therapy (rise from 420 to 980 mg/dl in three days) suggest that DIC was probably present.

During the second episode of septicemia, "relative hypofibrinogenemia" occurred with a fall in fibrinogen from 980 to 340 mg/dl. At this time the other coagulation tests indicated the presence of DIC.

Summary

DIC should be suspected when an acute, acquired hemorrhagic diathesis occurs in association with septicemia, hypotension or neoplasia. For early detection of DIC, the routine clinical examination of any critically ill patient should include specific inspection for signs of multisite bleeding, acral cyanosis and thrombosis. Blood loss in patients with DIC may be severe. The severity of bleeding should be carefully evaluated, and in particular, bleeding into the lungs or central nervous system considered. Patients with DIC can have many signs and symptoms but these are usually related to underlying disease states rather than to DIC.

CHAPTER V

COAGULATION STUDIES

DURING DIC THE PROTHROMBIN TIME, platelet count, and Fi titer are abnormal in 90 percent of patients, whereas the ELT, TT, and fibrinogen are abnormal in only 50 to 60 percent. The mean values for these tests are presented in Table I-I, and the individual data for each patient episode in Tables I-II and I-III. A bar graph depicts the range of results for each test during DIC (Fig. V-1).

CHANGES IN COAGULATION TEST VALUES ASSOCIATED WITH THE DEVELOPMENT OF DIC

We perform serial coagulation tests (PT, platelet counts and fibrinogen levels) daily when patients are suspected of having diseases that might acutely precipitate DIC. An average of six days will usually elapse from the onset of coagulation test abnormalities until the most abnormal levels are reached (Table V-I). When the coagulation tests reach levels that are scored as diagnostic (PT > 15 sec, platelet count < 150,000/ul and fibrinogen < 160 mg/dl), approximately 80 percent of the patients concurrently develop bleeding or thrombosis. Thus the coagulation test abnormalities parallel temporally the clinical symptoms. In addition, the average coagulation values change in the direction predicted by the diagnosis of DIC: rise in PT (5 sec prolongation), fall in platelets (−207,000/ul), and fall in fibrinogen (−224 mg/dl) (Table V-I). These changes represent dynamic evidence for the presence of DIC. When the diagnosis of DIC is difficult to establish by clinical criteria alone, comparison of serial coagulation values is of great aid.

CORRELATION OF COAGULATION ABNORMALITIES WITH CLINICAL STATES

Prognosis is highly correlated with the degree of abnormality of the coagulation tests at the time of diagnosis (Table

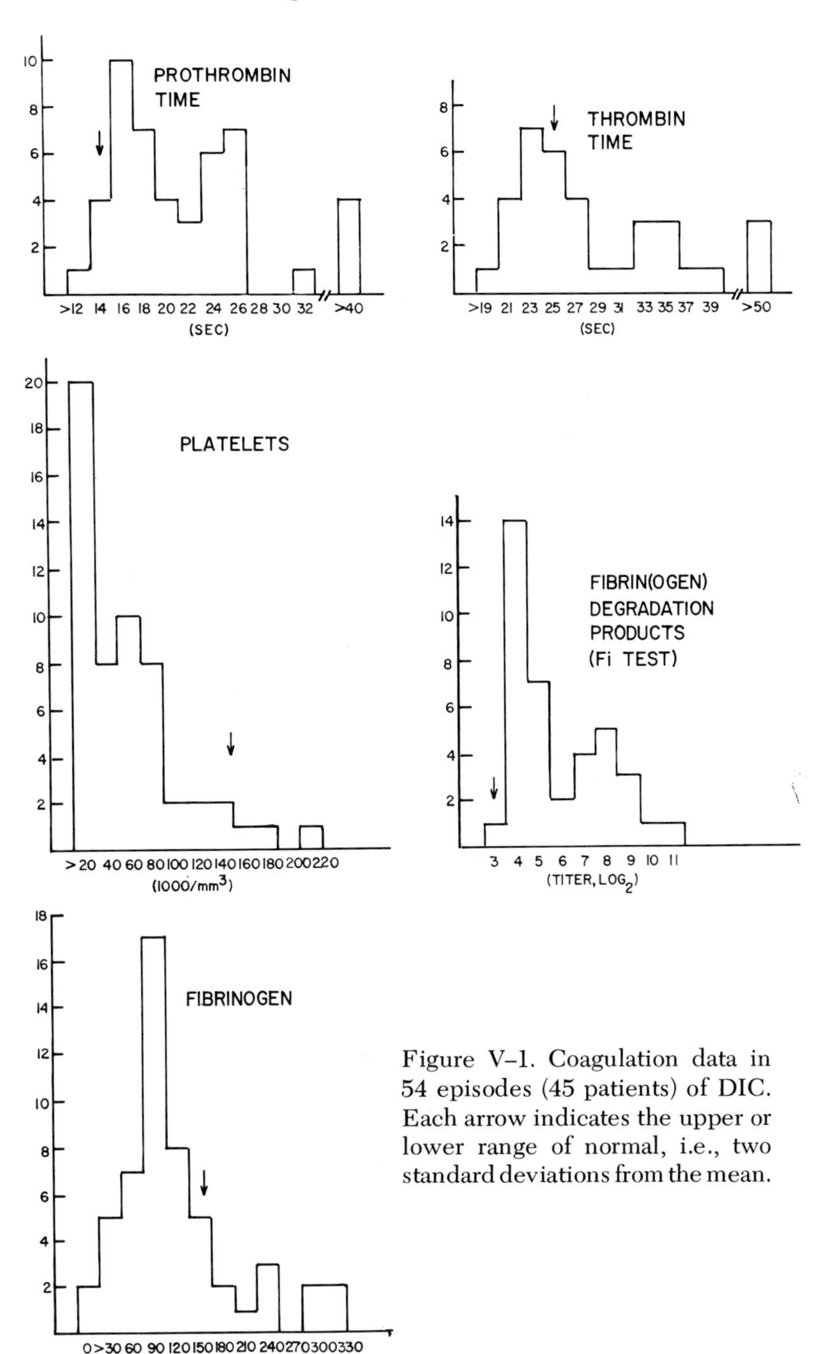

Figure V–1. Coagulation data in 54 episodes (45 patients) of DIC. Each arrow indicates the upper or lower range of normal, i.e., two standard deviations from the mean.

TABLE V-I
CHANGES IN COAGULATION VALUES
AS DIC APPEARS[1]

	Before DIC	*Change*	*Value During DIC*
PT (sec)	13.1 ± 2	+5.0	18.1
Platelet[2] (per ul)	257,000 ± 149,000	−207,000 ± 112,000	50,000 ± 50,000
Fibrinogen (mg/dl)	365 ± 195	−244 ± 157	121 ± 83
Time		5.8 ± 4.2 days	

[1] Calculated for 23 patients (PT 27 episodes, platelets 28 episodes, fibrinogen 23 episodes). Mean ± 1 SD.
[2] Excludes cases of leukemia; in cases of multiple episodes only initial episode included.

V-II). Patients who survived, whose bleeding stopped, and who subsequently had complete resolution of their underlying diseases had significantly less prolonged prothrombin times, higher platelet counts, and higher fibrinogen levels than the other patients.

Only a few other significant differences in coagulation test values are found among clinically distinguishable groups (Table V-II). In addition, there is little correlation of the degree of abnormality of one coagulation value with the degree of abnormality of another. However, when the ELT is abnormal, many of the coagulation test values correlate with one another (r maximally 0.74).

Bleeding severity is not correlated with the degree of abnormality of the coagulation tests. Likewise, underlying diseases are usually not correlated with these tests. Leukemia patients have the lowest platelet counts for obvious reasons. Of particular interest is the correlation of acral cyanosis, gram negative septicemia and hypotension with a higher fibrinogen and lower plasminogen level than are found in other patients with DIC. These functional changes may be explained by endotoxin stimulation of fibrinogen production (217) and endotoxin activation of factor XII, (and thus activation of the kallikrein and fibrinolytic systems) (*see* Chap. VIII).

Organ dysfunction is poorly correlated with degree of coagulation test abnormality. The only significant finding is more prolonged prothrombin times in patients with either pulmonary hemorrhage, pulmonary congestion, or coma.

TABLE V-II

CORRELATION OF CLINICAL STATES WITH COAGULATION TESTS

	LABORATORY												*CLINICAL*					
		During DIC							*After Therapy*									
	N	PT	Plat	Fib	Fi	ELT	TT	Plasminogen	PT	Plat	Fib	Fi	Overall Severity of Bleeding	# of Bleeding Sites	# of Transfusions	Hypotension	Length of Survival[1]	Survival (leave hospital)
Clinical Manifestations																		
Bleeding																		
None	8				−								×	×	×			+
Mild	14				+					+			×	×	×			
Moderate	17									+	++		×	×	×			−
Severe	15				−					−	− −		×	×	×			−
Local GI Bleeding	9			− −									+++	++	++			
Thrombosis																		
Severe Thrombi	9													−				
Severe Purpura	11												×				−	
Acrocyanosis	8			+				−−−			++					++		
Schistocytosis	14																	
Etiology																		
Neoplasia																		
Carcinoma	6								−									
Leukemia	7		−	−					−−−							−−		
Sepis																		
Gram-negative Septicemia	16			+											−	+	−	
Gram-positive Septicemia	6																−−	
Hypotension	27															×	−	
Acidosis																		
Organ Dysfunction																		
Pulmonary Dysfunction	34													++	+			
Hypoxemia	9							−−	−−−									
Pulmonary emboli	6							−	−−								−−	
Pulmonary hemorrhage	16	−											++	+++	+			−−
Pulmonary congestion	17	−												++			−−	
Renal Dysfunction	35							−								+		
Azotemia	18								−							+		

TABLE V-II
CORRELATION OF CLINICAL STATES WITH COAGULATION TESTS

		LABORATORY												*CLINICAL*					
		During DIC							*After Therapy*										
	N	PT	Plat	Fib	Fi	ELT	TT	Plasminogen	PT	Plat	Fib	Fi	Overall Severity of Bleeding	# of Bleeding Sites	# of Transfusions	Hypotension	Length of Survival[1]	Survival (leave hospital)
Oliguria	17									–	–						–	
Cardiac Dysfunction	25	–												+				
Cardiogenic shock syndrome	11													++		×		
Neurologic dysfunction	31													++		+++	–	––
Coma	18	–			–			–						++				
Diagnostic Tests																		
PT > 25 sec	16	×		–													––	
Plat < 25,000/μl	20		×	––														
Fibrinogen <100 mg/dl	22	–	–––	×						––								
Fi titer > 2^7	31				×							+					–	
+ ELT	22	–			(++)	×												
+ Thrombin Time	12						×											
Outcome																		
Died of bleeding or thrombosis	14	–								–	–		++					
Died during Episode of DIC	21	–		––					–	–			+	+			×	×
Survived	17	+	+	++						+	++							
Complete resolution of underlying disease	13	+	+	+++										–––				+++
Bleeding stopped	21	+	++	+++					++	++	++	++						++
Miscellaneous																		
Splenomegaly	10															++		
Steroid Therapy	19		––															
Vitamin K Therapy	15	–	––										++	+++				

Symbols indicate the occurrence of significant differences between the indicated patient groups and the remainder of the patients: Blank, no significant difference; ×, part of the criteria for selecting the patient group; + or –, $P < 0.05$; ++ or ––, $P < 0.01$; +++ or –––, $P < 0.001$. The + symbols indicate a higher or more normal laboratory value, while – symbols indicate the opposite. In the case of clinical observations + symbols indicate: more severe bleeding, greater number of bleeding sites, more units transfused, a higher incidence of hypotension, longer duration or higher incidence of survival while – symbols indicate the opposite.

[1] Patients surviving to leave the hospital were excluded.

Summary

The prothrombin time becomes prolonged, platelet count falls, and fibrinogen level decreases as patients develop DIC. These simultaneous changes are strongly diagnostic of DIC in the individual patient. The degree of coagulation test abnormalities at the time of diagnosis of DIC is related to survival and cessation of bleeding but in only a few instances to other clinical phenomena.

CHAPTER VI

SYSTEMIC FIBRINOLYSIS

THE ROLE OF SYSTEMIC FIBRINOLYSIS (pathologic proteolysis) in DIC has been a subject of debate in the literature. Much of the discussion centers about a definition of systemic fibrinolysis, the tests necessary for its diagnosis, and the relation between systemic fibrinolysis and DIC. The clinical importance of this controversy is that systemic fibrinolysis, if present alone, would be treated with EACA, a drug that inhibits fibrinolysis by blocking activation of plasminogen to plasmin (3). However, if the systemic fibrinolysis is secondary to DIC, EACA used alone could precipitate thrombotic complications (76,119,141). Thrombosis would occur if the fibrinolysis were a compensatory mechanism acting to lyse the intravascular clots formed by DIC.

Systemic fibrinolysis is defined as the presence of pathological proteolysis due to the action of plasmin in the systemic circulation. Currently, the ELT*, which measures plasminogen activators, is the most sensitive and easily performed test for systemic fibrinolysis available in a clinical hematologic laboratory. Immediate lysis of a euglobulin clot probably reflects a highly activated fibrinolytic system capable of immediate dissolution of any newly formed fibrin thrombus (*see* history of Case 30 below).

CASE 30 (TABLE VI-I)—RETAINED DEAD FETUS AND SYSTEMIC FIBRINOLYSIS: A 27-year-old woman (gravid I, para 0) entered for dilation and curettage of a retained dead fetus. At five months gestation vaginal bleeding occurred and during the ensuing two months the uterus failed to enlarge. At operation, necrotic placental

* It has been claimed that the ELT test as performed by the method of Kowalski *et al.* (99) is not valid unless fibrinogen is added to the test mixture (16). For reasons stated in Chapter II, we believe that the ELT is a function of multiple factors. Although we have not added fibrinogen as a routine procedure, four of the patients had normal fibrinogen levels of 160 to 350 mg/dl, suggesting that factors other than fibrinogen alone are responsible for an abnormal ELT. No correlation existed in this series between the fibrinogen level and an abnormal ELT (*see* Chap. XII).

tissue was removed; no amniotic fluid was seen. Four units of oxytocin were given and the estimated blood loss was 50 cc.

One hour later, she suddenly became hypotensive, apneic, and no blood pressure could be obtained. The arterial pH was 7.20. Ephedrine, four units of packed RBC and isoproterinol were given; the blood pressure rose to 100 systolic, 50 diastolic, the pulse to 140, and spontaneous respirations reappeared. EKG showed an acute infero-posterior myocardial infarct, first degree A-V block, and atrial and ventricular bigeminy. She was comatose with a right gaze palsy and marked acral cyanosis. Oliguria, vaginal bleeding, hematemesis, and hematuria appeared. The tests of clotting function were strikingly abnormal including a plasminogen level of 0.5 units/ml (Tables VI-I and VIII-III).

During the first day, she received sodium bicarbonate, packed red cells and albumin. By 48 hours all bleeding stopped and the acral cyanosis was gone. By 72 hours all tests of clotting function were normal. Gradually the neurologic signs cleared, and serial EKG and enzymes showed an evolving myocardial infarct. Upon discharge from the hospital one month later, no sequelae were present.

Comment: This case of DIC and secondary systemic fibrinolysis occurred as a result of uterine curettage for a retained dead fetus. The history suggests that necrotic tissue debris with tissue thromboplastin was introduced into the maternal vascular system, with implantation into many maternal organs, including the brain and heart (105, 158). The consequence was DIC, amniotic fluid emboli with the various observed forms of organ dysfunction.

Systemic fibrinolysis was indicated by the immediate ELT, high FDP titer, and low plasminogen level. As the platelet count was initially only slightly lower (129,000 to 144,000/ul) than the lower

TABLE VI-I
CASE 30

	PT (sec)	Platelet count (per ul)	Fibrinogen (mg/dl)	PTT (sec)	ELT (min)	Fi
Pre-op		"normal"	240			
Post-op D&C						
+ 4 hr	28	129,000		55	Immed	1:512
+ 8 hr	20	144,000	167	34	5	1:32
+ 11 hr	17	96,000	192	35	>120	
+ 24 hr	16	93,000	170			
+ 48 hr	12	121,000	240	35	>120	1:16
+ 3 day	12	139,000				
+ 5 day	12	257,000				
+ 14 day	12	405,000				

range of normal, some would have classified the patient as having primary fibrinolysis. However, a further fall in platelet count occurred subsequently, indicating consumption of platelets (and hence the presence of DIC) in addition to pathological proteolysis. The delay in platelet count fall observed occasionally, and the slow rise occurring over a two-week period is typical of the response seen in DIC. The change in the ELT from immediate to 5 minutes to normal during a seven hour interval suggests that rapid changes in the fibrinolytic system were taking place.

This patient also illustrates that once the inciting mechanisms of DIC can be removed, resolution takes place and heparin therapy may not be required.

A second useful test is determination of the level of plasma plasminogen itself. Since only liver disease causes a decrease of this precursor, a fall is suggestive of systemic or widespread fibrinolysis. Since tests for FDP, such as the Fi, SCT, TRCHII may reflect the digestion of fibrin at multiple local sites or fibrin(ogen)olysis in the systemic circulation, their results cannot be regarded as absolute indicators of a systemic process. Whole blood clot lysis is useful when present but occurs relatively infrequently (< 5%); also it is insensitive because of the presence of normally occurring plasmin inhibitors (185).

The majority of episodes of DIC are not associated with systemic fibrinolysis. Thus, abnormal ELTs were observed in fewer than a fifth of the patients in this series and in the literature (130). Although a short ELT can be observed on occasion as an isolated finding in normal individuals (97), other coagulation test data indicate the presence of a hemostatic abnormality (Table VI-II). Some underlying diseases in which the ELT has been abnormal are listed in Table VI-III. This list may eventually contain all diseases capable of precipitating DIC.

Rank order correlations and chi square analysis disclose a relation between the ELT and the titer of FDP. The average Fi titer with a positive ELT was 1:160, while the Fi titer was only 1:32 when the ELT was negative ($p < 0.005$). Further, the Fi titer was always above 1:30 (average 1:256) when the ELT was immediate, while the Fi titer was as low as 1:16 when the ELT was abnormally short, but greater than immediate.

TABLE VI-II
COAGULATION DATA IN SYSTEMIC FIBRINOLYSIS

ELT (min)	Fi	Plasminogen (casein u.)	TT (sec)	PT (sec)	Platelet count (per ul)	Fibrinogen (mg/dl)	Patient (episode)
Immed	1:512	0.50	56	28	129,000	167	30
Immed	1:512	0.50	ND	109	49,000	**	20
Immed	1:160	1.94	35	25	69,000	40	2
Immed	1:128	ND	86	47	147,000	240	24
Immed	1:80	ND	ND	29	19,000	160	28
3	1:256	1.43	ND	31	14,000	96	33a
5	1:16	3.43	ND	15	180,000	350	15
5	1:16	1.66	33	43	12,000	80	41
10	1:1280	2.25	26	18	65,000	74	13a
15	1:128	1.08	36	21	20,000	34	35b
55	1:64	ND	27	25	91,000	89	37
90	1:2560	ND	90	20	52,000	94	13b
> 120	1:8	5.50 ± 1.8	20 ±1.6	11.5 ±1.0	250,000 ±50,000	230 ±35	Normal values ±1 S.D.

** Incoagulable plasma   Immed—Immediate   ND—Not done

A question frequently raised is whether systemic fibrinolysis is primary or whether it is secondary to DIC. In experimentally produced primary systemic fibrinolysis in humans, the platelet count remains normal (59). Thus, the preservation of a normal platelet count has been cited as evidence of systemic fibrinolysis occurring without DIC (16). However, if serial platelet counts are performed in patients with abnormal ELTs, a fall in platelet count can usually be detected, indicating the consumption of clotting elements in addition to pathologic proteolysis. A delay in platelet count fall is sometimes seen in DIC and this delay may explain some of the "normal platelet counts" with systemic fibrinolysis previously noted.

Three patients in this study had abnormal ELTs and normal

TABLE VI-III
DISEASES ASSOCIATED WITH SYSTEMIC FIBRINOLYSIS

Tissue injury	
Obstetrical	1
Surgical	1
Neoplastic	
Prostatic carcinoma	2
Granulocytic leukemia	2
Endothelial injury	
Bacterial septicemia	3
Viremia	1
Reticuloendothelial system injury	
Liver injury	1

platelet counts or platelet counts that were initially just below normal. In one (*see* history of Case 15 in Chap. XI) treatment with EACA resulted in catastrophic thrombosis and unmasking of DIC; in another (*see* history of Case 24 in Chap. IV) thrombocytopenia subsequently developed and heparin therapy was associated with clinical and coagulation test improvement (*see also* Case 30 above). Lastly in five of six patients with abnormal ELTs, fibrin thrombi were found at autopsy, a feature not encountered in experimental animal models of systemic primary fibrinolysis (58). Thus we always found systemic fibrinolysis to be associated with DIC.

Additional clinical evidence also suggests that systemic fibrinolysis is secondary to DIC. As the DIC abated in five patients who were treated without EACA, major bleeding ceased and signs of systemic fibrinolysis (abnormal ELT, Fi titer) also disappeared (Fig. VI-2) (174). This is particularly reinforced in the following patient who had multiple episodes of clinically significant DIC and systemic fibrinolysis.

CASE 13 (FIG. VI-1)—PROSTATIC CARCINOMA AND SYSTEMIC FIBRINOLYSIS: A 69 year-old white male entered for hematuria. One month before, spontaneous ecchymoses appeared over the skin. Three weeks later examination revealed a hard prostatic nodule. The hematocrit was 35%, acid phosphatase 9.0 units, platelets 82,000/ul, and PT 18 sec. The ecchymoses increased in number, he developed a traumatic hemarthrosis of the ankle, and on the day of admission he urinated gross blood.

Examination revealed multiple ecchymoses scattered over the entire body, with no petechiae, thromboses or palpable purpura. A hard unilateral prostatic mass extended into both seminal vesicles. Enlarged inguinal and axillary nodes and a large 10 × 10 cm epigastric and left flank mass were detected. The hematocrit was 34% and WBC 6900. The tests of clotting function were markedly abnormal and included an ELT of 10 minutes, Fi 1:1280, and plasminogen 2.3 u/ml. (Fig. VI-2). X-rays revealed extensive osteolytic involvement of the lumbo-sacral spine. Bone marrow biopsy revealed metastatic prostatic carcinoma. Heparin (6000 U every 4 hr) was administered and during the ensuing four days, all bleeding stopped and each laboratory test of hemostasis, except the platelet count, returned significantly towards normal.

Tumor chemotherapy with conjugated estrogens (20 mg IV for 2 doses) and then stilbestrol (5 mg oral, twice daily) was begun. Two days later, the tests of clotting function were again very abnor-

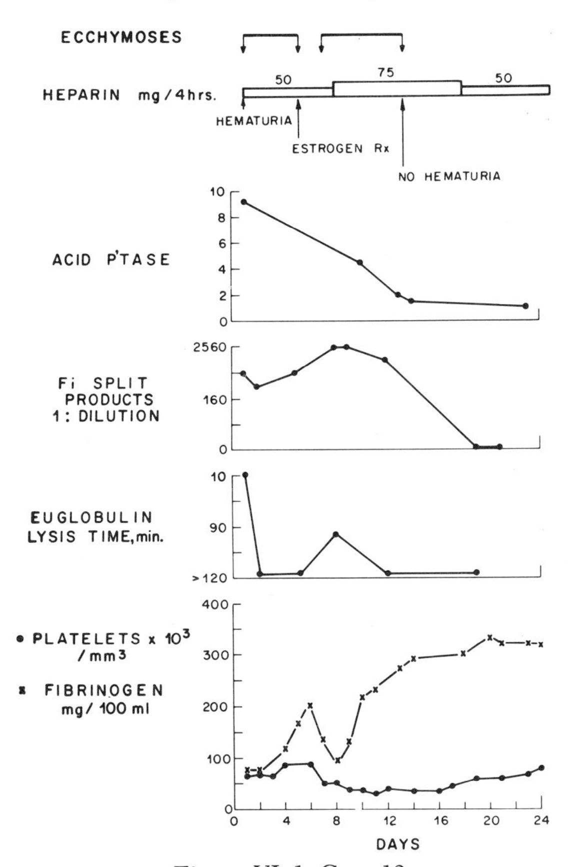

Figure VI–1. Case 13

mal and included an ELT of 90 minutes, Fi 1:2560 and plasminogen 2.6 u/ml. Because the whole blood clotting time had dropped to low normal, dosage of heparin was increased to 75 mg IV every four hours; the whole blood clotting time returned to high therapeutic levels. Within three days all tests of clotting function showed a partial return towards normal; except the platelet count. Radiotherapy was given subsequently and on the twenty-third day the heparin was stopped. The Fi titer was normal.

On the thirtieth hospital day the Fi rose to 1:640. The tests of clotting function were again mildly abnormal. One day later ecchymoses appeared on the dorsum and plantar aspect of the feet and toes. Then the right leg suddenly became cold and blue. Pulses from the femoral area distally could not be obtained. Heparin (6000 U every 4 hr) was begun. Gradually the leg became warm and the femoral and foot pulses returned. For the remainder of the

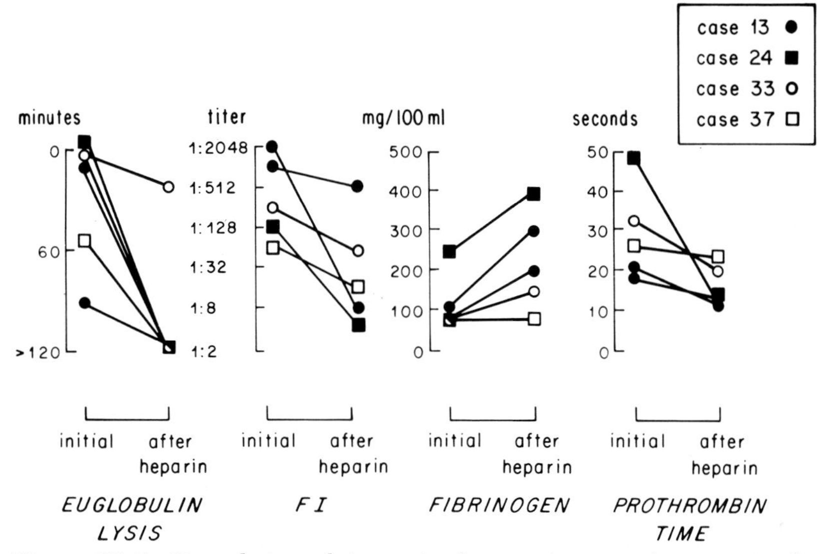

Figure VI–2. Coagulation changes in four patients with systemic fibrinolysis after heparin therapy.

hospital course, heparin was given. The PT remained normal, platelets 95,000–180,000/ul, fibrinogen 260–390 mg/dl. The patient was discharged on the fifty-sixth hospital day with a Fi of 1:80.

Comment: Because of the short ELT (10 min), low plasminogen levels, very elevated Fi titer (1:2560), and modest thrombocytopenia (100,000/ul), this patient might easily have been classified as an example of primary fibrinolysis. However, with heparin therapy alone, the bleeding ceased and the laboratory evidence of fibrinolysis disappeared. This patient also illustrates how the cytolytic effect of estrogens on tumor cells can precipitate DIC and how the dosage of heparin sometimes must be raised coincident with cancer chemotherapy. Finally, the chronic nature of tumor induced DIC is evident. After the heparin therapy was terminated the Fi rose from 1:10 to 1:640 and by the time of discharge had stabilized at 1:80.

Summary

The study of eleven patients with systemic fibrinolysis suggests that systemic fibrinolysis occurs in DIC, an abnormal ELT is not a manifestation of low fibrinogen levels alone, high titers of FDP may in part be due to systemic fibrinolysis, and systemic fibrinolysis is a complication of DIC and probably does not occur as an isolated “primary” entity.

CHAPTER VII

HEMATOLOGIC MANIFESTATIONS

PERIPHERAL BLOOD

Red Blood Cells

PATIENTS WITH DIC ARE USUALLY anemic (average hematocrit 29%). The most common causes are acute blood loss and impaired red cell production. The loss that occurs in the gastrointestinal tract is frequently recognized. However, two to three units of blood can be lost over a several day period from venipuncture, wound sites, or large subcutaneous hematomas before the importance of such sites is recognized.

Impaired red cell production is common in patients with DIC because of the underlying diseases. Examples include marrow suppression by acute and chronic sepsis or uremia, marrow infiltration by leukemia or other neoplastic processes, toxic effects of drugs and vitamin deficiency, particularly folic acid, during prolonged periods of parenteral feedings. One expression of impaired production that we noted uniformly was the lack of erythroid hyperplasia in bone marrow specimens despite the presence of anemia, hypoxia and acute blood loss.

Clinically significant hemolysis was rarely observed in our patients. In Chapter I evidence is presented from the literature that hemolysis can initiate DIC (109) probably in part by the release of phospholipid (123). The general mechanisms involved include destruction of red cells by parasitic organisms, e.g., malaria (Table XII-II, Case xiii) (41), vascular lesions (15) release of stroma from the red cell (10), and fragmentation of red cells (schistocytosis) on fibrin strands (Fig. VII-1, *see* Chap. X) (19,172,176).

Although some evidence for hemolysis was found in about one-fifth of patients with DIC, severe hemolysis is infrequent.

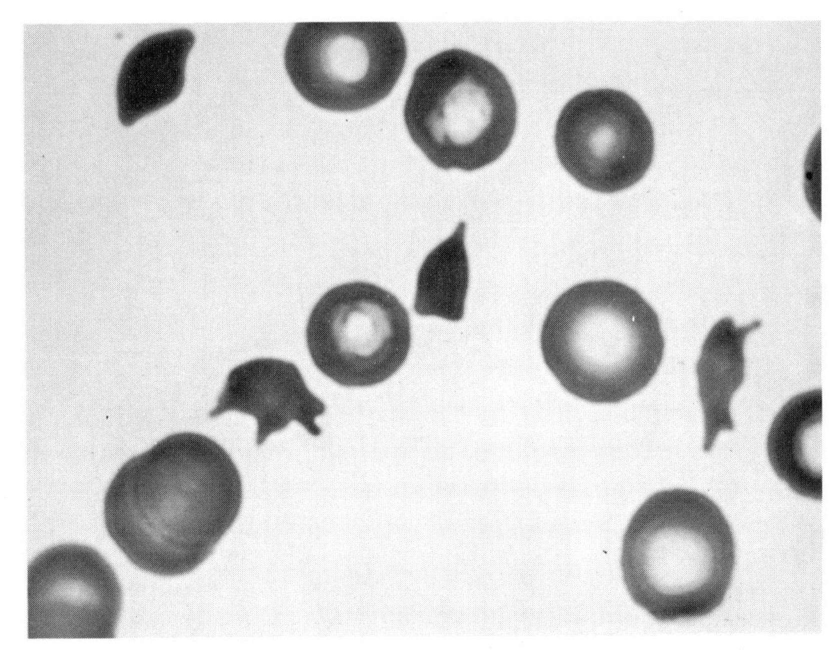

Figure VII–1. Schistocytes. Case 28. (Wright stain × 2150).

Little correlation exists among the degree of schistocytosis and the degree of coagulation test abnormalities, reticulocyte count, hematocrit, or bilirubin levels. Although in some cases the schistocytosis might be an effect of DIC, it is important to realize that in many cases hemolysis, schistocytosis, and DIC can be traced to an underlying disease process affecting blood vessels (e.g., systemic aspergillosis). Table VII-I presents sample data for eight patients in whom hemolysis was suspected.

White Blood Cells

The majority of patients who do not have leukemia demonstrate marked leukocytosis (average WBC 20,500/ul). A neutrophilic leukocytosis with an increased number of young myeloid cells (shift to the left) is the usual finding. Bone marrow examination in these patients also discloses a marked myeloid hyperplasia, with a moderate but orderly shift to young cells. These changes appear related to the underlying primary diseases that stress the marrow, such as sepsis.

TABLE VII-I
HEMOLYSIS

Patient #	Schistocytosis	HCT	Reticulocyte count (%)	Nucleated RBC/100 WBC	Total units blood transf.	Clinically evident bleeding	Thrombi	Comment
Hemolysis, probably related to DIC								
28	4 +	23	9.8	32	15	brisk	+	Aspergillosis Serum hemoglobin 23.3 mg /dl
17	4 +	29	0.6	1	3	brisk	–	↓ haptoglobin
45	2 +	30	1.4	1	8	brisk	+	Aspergillosis ↓ haptoglobin
8	2 +	23	6.8	0	6	oozing	+	Folic acid deficiency
Hemolysis, not related to DIC								
34	1 +	20–30	9–20	0	20	none	–	Coombs + hemolytic anemia before DIC
Doubtful hemolysis								
26	2 +	23	2.4	0	0	oozing	+	Acral gangrene
36	1 +	30	3.2	0	3	none	+	Acral gangrene
6	0	26	5.9	0	5	oozing	+	Purpura fulminans iron deficiency ↓ urine urobilinogen

Platelets

The thrombocytopenia of DIC is usually apparent in the examination of the peripheral blood smear. Fifty-two percent of patients had platelet counts below 50,000/ul, while 37 percent had counts below 20,000/ul. Examination of the bone marrow in nonleukemic patients disclosed decreased to normal numbers of megakaryocytes; increased numbers were not observed although peripheral destruction is probably the major mechanism of platelet loss in DIC. Suppression of bone marrow thrombopoiesis by sepsis (157) and drugs (*see* history of Case 1) probably play a role in the generation of the severe thrombocytopenia.

CASE 1—THROMBOCYTOPENIA, WITH SEPTICEMIA, DRUG TOXICITY AND DIC: A 58 year-old female had a cup arthroplasty for degenerative hip disease, complicated by recurrent pulmonary embolism, atrial fibrillation, and pulmonary congestion. Heparin (6000 U every 4 hr) and digitalis were given. The initial platelet count was 306,000/ul and rose to 554,000/ul. On the thirteenth day pulmonary embolism again occurred (while on heparin) and the inferior vena cava was ligated. Warfarin was begun and one week later the PT was 18 sec, platelet count 1,133,000/ul and fibrinogen 456 mg/dl. Heparin and warfarin were then stopped.

On the thirty-eighth day serratia septicemia and a subhepatic abscess developed from a perforated gallbladder. Surgical drainage was performed and chloramphenicol (3 gm/day) given. On the fiftieth day the platelet count was 26,000/ul, PT 13 sec, fibrinogen 210 mg/dl and PTT 30 sec. Because chloramphenicol toxicity was suspected, the therapy was discontinued. Over the next six days the platelet count rose to 136,000/ul.

On the fifty-sixth day she was febrile and multiple blood cultures continued to show serratia. Kanamycin was started. Helmet cells and occasional burr cells were present in the peripheral blood smear. A laparotomy was required to drain a left subdiaphragmatic abscess infected with serratia. The platelet count fell to 36,000/ul. Blood cultures continued to grow out serratia and she became disoriented, tachypneic and developed an acute antero-lateral subendocardial infarct. On the sixty-sixth day profuse bleeding from the mouth, trachea, rectum and venipuncture sites suddenly appeared. The PT was 17 sec, platelet count 9000/ul, fibrinogen 108 mg/dl, PTT 49 sec, TT 27 sec, ELT normal. The hematocrit fell from 35% to 18%. Heparin (6000 U every 4 hr), fibrinogen (6 gm), platelets (4 units) and whole blood were given. The bleeding stopped promptly. The fibrinogen rose to 250 mg/dl and remained above

200 mg/dl for the three days until death. The platelets and PT did not change. No autopsy was performed.

Comment: This complicated case illustrates the differential diagnosis of three instances of rising or falling platelet counts. Initially, the platelets rose from 306,000 to 1,133,000/ul and may represent a rebound phenomenon after heparin was given for pulmonary embolism. The second episode was chloramphenicol-induced thrombocytopenia. The diagnosis was established by the normal PT and fibrinogen, and a prompt rise in the platelet count once chloramphenicol therapy was terminated. The third and terminal episode of thrombocytopenia represented DIC triggered by serratia septicemia.

BONE MARROW EXAMINATION

The major findings on examination of bone marrow specimens (aspirate, biopsy, or autopsy) have been mentioned: myeloid hyperplasia with a shift to young forms; usually normal or decreased erythroid precursors and megakaryocytes. Bone marrow aspiration is well tolerated by patients with DIC despite the patients' acquired hemorrhagic diathesis. Fibrin thrombi were rarely seen in marrow section even at autopsy and thus bone marrow examination is of little aid in the diagnosis of DIC. However, the examination appears indicated when the cause of severe leukopenia, thrombocytopenia or anemia is unexplained. The not uncommon finding of megaloblastosis and neoplasia and the fact that marrow can be cultured argue for the usefulness of this examination as a diagnostic aid.

CHAPTER VIII

KALLIKREIN SYSTEM

THE BIOCHEMICAL PATHOGENESIS OF DIC can vary, depending upon the underlying disease (Fig. I-1). Distinction between the various pathways may be difficult if judged by usual assays of blood coagulation factors. Simultaneous thrombin and plasmin activation result in complex and sometimes inconsistent changes in factor levels. The significance of elevated levels of inactive coagulation factors is unknown and reliable assays for most activated factors are unavailable. In addition, *in vitro* systems do not necessarily mirror *in vivo* changes since activated clotting factors may be cleared by the liver (43) and this defense mechanism may be compromised in liver disease.

One biochemical pathway, which involves the activation of factor XII, is subject to laboratory confirmation. When factor XII (Hageman factor) is activated, it (143) or its derivatives (88) are known to convert prekallikrein into the proteolytic enzyme kallikrein. Kallikrein exhibits arginine esterase activity, forming the basis of a biochemical assay for kallikrein, its precursor prekallikrein and its inhibitor, kallikrein inhibitor (31–3). The assay measures the development of tosyl arginine esterase (TAMe) activity as a function of time under controlled conditions of ionic strength and pH after exposure to kaolin. The reaction specificity can be confirmed by examining the substrate specificity of several methyl esters, such as benzoyl arginine (BAMe), tosyl lysine (TLMe), and acetyl lysine (ALMe), and comparing them to tosyl arginine (TAMe).

The activation of Hageman factor produces a characteristic pattern of plasma kallikrein activation. A transient increase in spontaneous tosyl arginine esterase activity with the substrate specificity of purified plasma kallikrein is followed by depletion of prekallikrein and disappearance of kallikrein inhibitor (81,128), the latter two forming inactive stochiometric complexes having no activity (68). Not only is prekallikrein activation a potential useful probe for elucidating one site of initiation of DIC, but kallikrein formation also has important functional consequences. Kallikrein releases bradykinin from the plasma alpha 2 globulin, kininogen. Bradykinin, besides mimicking many characteristics of the inflammatory response (91), is the most potent mammalian vasodepressor substance known. Thus hypotension might be expected to occur in diseases associated with Hageman factor activation. The application of kallikrein analysis is well illustrated in the following patient with fatal meningococcemia (128).

CASE 20—FULMINANT MENINGOCOCCEMIA AND WATERHOUSE-FRIEDERICKSEN SYNDROME IN A PREGNANT WOMAN: A 24-year-old woman was admitted with fever and petechiae. One day before she developed a sore throat, tender cervical lymphadenopathy, fever and malaise. One hour before admission petechiae appeared. On physical examination the pulse was 140, temperature 104°F, and blood pressure 70 by palpation. Extensive petechiae and purpura were noted. She was alert without nuchal rigidity. The remainder of the examination was unremarkable. Vaginal bleeding then developed and was accompanied by the expulsion of a normal 2 cm fetus.

Examination of the cerebrospinal fluid showed two to three lymphocytes and normal protein and glucose concentration. Culture of blood and cerebrospinal fluid grew abundant *Neisseria meningitidis* in pure culture, as did a throat culture from the previous day. The hematocrit was 45%, and WBC 16,000/ul with a shift to the left. Coagulation screening tests showed a PT of 105 sec, platelet count 68,000/ul, fibrinogen 0 mg/dl, Fi titer 1:512, factor V 7%, factor VIII 12% and factor X 50%. Kallikrein data is presented in Figure VIII-1. Penicillin, heparin (6250 U), oxytocin, digoxin, plasma, oxygen, and morphine were begun, but she died within 3 hours.

Autopsy showed diffuse hemorrhages in adrenals, skin, and lungs. Scattered fibrin thrombi were present in the small vessels of many organs. The uterus, the expelled fetus, and the placenta were unremarkable.

Comment: The findings are those of overwhelming meningococcal septicemia, severe hypotension, and DIC with secondary fibrinolysis.

The data for the components of the kallikrein system in Case 20 are shown in the middle curve of Figure VIII-1 and

IN VIVO ACTIVATION OF KALLIKREN SYSTEM

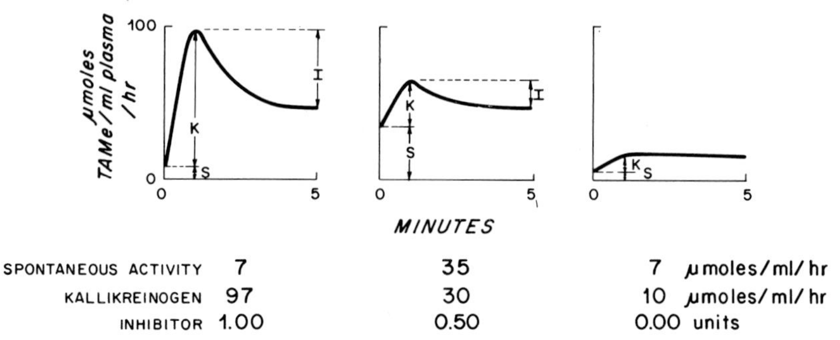

Figure VIII–1. Comparison of an assay curve from normal subjects with curves early and late in the in vivo activation of plasma kallikrein. The assay curve constructed from the mean of 36 normal subjects is on the left. The center curve is from a woman who died three hours after admission to the hospital with acute fulminant meningococcemia (case 20), while the right curve was obtained 24 hours after the onset of a streptococcal septicemia (case 37). Calculated values below each curve are for spontaneous activity (S), kallikreinogen (now prekallikrein) (K), and kallikrein inhibitor (I). (Mason, Kleeberg, Dolan, and Colman: *Ann Int Med, 73:* 545, 1970).

is compared with a normal population (left) and a patient in bacteremic shock of over one day's duration (right). Compared with normal persons the spontaneous activity in Case 20 was increased while the prekallikrein and kallikrein inhibitors were decreased. The factor XII levels were also decreased to 23 percent of normal. Both the levels of prekallikrein and kallikrein inhibitors fell further in the patient who was in prolonged shock.

The elevated spontaneous activity in Case 20 was compared with known plasma esterases by determining its relative activity against several methyl esters (Table VIII-I). These ratios are similar to those of purified human plasma kallikrein and unlike those of other related plasma esterases such as thrombin, plasmin, and the esterolytic activity of the first component of complement (31).

The entire profile of the kallikrein system in this patient is what would be expected if DIC were initiated by factor XII activation (222). The hypotension may be in part related to kallikrein release of bradykinin. The entire process is prob-

TABLE VIII-I

RELATIVE ACTIVITIES AGAINST VARIOUS SUBSTRATES OF A PLASMA ESTRASE IN A SEPTIC PATIENT AND PURIFIED PLASMA ENZYMES

	BAMe	TLMe	ALMe	TAMe
DIC and *N. meningitidis* septicemia (Case 20)	0.92	0.49	0.49	1.00
Purified plasma enzymes				
Kallikrein	0.85	0.31	0.37	1.00
Thrombin	1.00	1.70	0.40	1.00
Plasmin	1.01	1.48	2.35	1.00
C_1	1.03	1.50	2.33	1.00

(Mason and Colman: *Thromb Diathes Haemor 26*:325, 1971)

ably related to endothelial damage with consequent exposure of subendothelial collagen to Hageman factor.

The exact role of bradykinin release in causing shock in septicemia is unclear. Endotoxin-induced shock in experimental animals produces endothelial damage (67,114), kinin release, and, in monkeys, hemodynamic changes similar to bacteremic shock in man (147). Most likely bradykinin plays a role in the early phase of septicemic hypotension but the consequences of poor tissue perfusion, e.g. acidosis, serve to perpetuate the low blood pressure. Thus, the activation by endotoxin of the kallikrein-kinin system observed *in vivo* may be mediated through endothelial damage leading to factor XII activation.

Twenty-three of 45 patients with DIC in this series were studied and showed a mild increase in mean spontaneous activity (which may represent kallikrein) and a mild decrease in mean prekallikrein, kallikrein inhibitor and Hageman factor (Tables VIII-II, VIII-III). Compared to normals, patients classified as having endothelial injury (including septicemia with gram negative, gram positive organisms or viremia) had increased spontaneous esterolytic activity (kallikrein) and decreased prekallikrein, kallikrein inhibitor and factor XII. Thus, DIC in these patients is probably initiated by factor XII activation. In contrast, patients with tissue injury (usually malignancy), where thromboplastin release may be the initiating agent, showed no changes in the kallikrein system. Too

TABLE VIII-II

PLASMA KALLIKREIN ACTIVITY AND HAGEMAN FACTOR IN DIC

Patient Group	N	Spontaneous Activity	Prekallikrein	Kallikrein Inhibitor	Hageman Factor
		μ moles TAMe/ml/hr[1]		units[2]	% of normal[3]
Normal	36	7 ± 4	97 ± 24	0.99 ± 0.17	98 ± 18
DIC, all patients	23	11	61	0.73	62
DIC with					
Tissue injury[4]	10	9	82	0.83	75
Endothelial injury[5]	11	14	40	0.41	57
Platelet or red cell injury[6]	2	6	44	1.12	N.D.
Liver disease[7]	6				
Septicemia	4	9	22	0.39	53
Non-septicemic	2	6	77	1.14	N.D.
Normotensive	10	9	53	0.72	61
Hypotensive[8]	13				
Blood loss	4	9	99	1.11	100
Septicemia	9	14	56	0.57	56
Gram negative	6	17	41	0.35	50

[1] Micromoles of TAMe hydrolyzed per ml plasma (mean ± 1 SD). Spontaneous activity represents zero time esterolytic activity; prekallikrein represents activity 1 minute after exposure to kaolin (peak value). Spontaneous esterase activity had the same ester substrate ratios as purified human plasma kallikrein towards a variety of substituted basic amino acid substrates when compared with TAMe.

[2] Kallikrein inhibitor unit is defined as a 50% decrease of TAMe μmoles hydrolyzed between 1 and 5 minutes after kaolin exposure (mean ± 1 SD).

[3] Assay performed by a modification of the partial thromboplastin time assay using congenitally deficient substrates (mean ± 1 SD) (Ref. 198).

[4] Cases 30, 15, 12, 13A, 2, 5, 16A, 21, 27, 35A.

[5] Cases 1, 3, 10A, 14, 20, 36, 40, 31, 37, 17, 33A.

[6] Cases 6A, 34.

[7] Cases 10, 33, 35, 37 (septic); 6, 40 (non-septic).

[8] Cases 12, 15, 30, 35A (blood loss); 1, 3, 14, 17, 20, 31, 33A, 36, 40 (septicemia).

TABLE VIII-III
PLASMA KALLIKREIN ACTIVITY AND HAGEMAN FACTOR IN 23 PATIENTS WITH DIC

Patient Group	Case #	Spontaneous Activity μ moles TAMe/ml/hr	Prekallikrein μ moles TAMe/ml/hr	Kallikrein Inhibitor units	Hageman Factor % of normal
Tissue injury					
Obstetrical	30	11	116	1.15	
Surgery, extensive	15	9	70	0.73	
Neoplasia					
Prostate	12	8	104	1.28	100
	13A	13	102	0.95	
Leukemia	2	17	90	0.58	100
	5	10	104	0.98	
	16A	5	44	0.54	53
	21	6	54	0.68	45
	27	9	30	0.65	80
Hemorrhagic, shock	35A	6	106	1.28	
Endothelial injury					
Gram negative septicemia	1	7	53	1.05	50
	1, 24 hrs	9	51	0.72	
	3	7	65	0.35	42
	3, 24 hrs	12	66	0.62	
	3, 72 hrs	13	34	0.03	
	10A	7	11	0.59	
	14	18	51	0.56	
	14, 24 hrs	13	47	0.61	
	14, 48 hrs	19	32	0.26	
	20	35	30	0.50	23
	36	14	78	0.60	100
	40	9	67	0.98	
Gram positive septicemia	31	12	77	0.65	81
	37	7	10	0.00	65
Viremia	17	14	74	0.75	
	33A	11	9	0.00	
	33A, 48 hrs	13	6	0.00	41
Platelet or red cell injury					
Purpura fulminans	6A	6	48	1.00	
Coombs + hem.	34	7	41	1.25	25
Normal		7 ± 4	97 ± 24	0.99 ± 17	98 ± 18

few patients with platelet or red cell injury have been studied as yet. In addition, patients with septicemia and hypotension showed evidence of factor XII activation as opposed to normotensive patients or patients with hypotension due to blood loss (128). Patients with septicemia but without hypotension had neither DIC nor kallikrein activation (128). When DIC developed in patients with liver disease, only those with concomitant septicemia had kallikrein activation.

Thus, determination of a factor XII activated system allows insight into one mechanism activating DIC. The development of an antibody to tissue thromboplastin (145) will allow delineation of another triggering mechanism of DIC. It is hoped that identification of the specific pathogenetic mechanisms initiating DIC in the individual patient will allow for design of more specific modes of therapy.

CHAPTER IX

ORGAN DYSFUNCTION

MOST PATIENTS WITH DIC demonstrate signs of impaired function of at least one major organ system; in many cases, several organ systems show impaired function simultaneously. Although it has been suggested (116) that DIC precipitates widespread symptoms and signs of dysfunction of multiple organs, in our experience the majority of such symptoms and signs are related to pathophysiologic mechanisms other than DIC (*see also* "Signs and Symptoms" in Chap. IV). The two major exceptions are patients with hemorrhage into the lungs or central nervous system.

CARDIAC DYSFUNCTION

Many patients had clinical evidence of cardiac dysfunction manifested by: acute ischemia, arrhythmia or conduction defects (demonstrated by electrocardiogram); pulmonary congestion detected by X-ray; syndrome of "cardiogenic shock" (elevated central venous pressure, hypotension, pulmonary congestion and oliguria); or embolic phenomenon arising from the heart, confirmed pathologically (see Table IV-V). Although twenty-six patients (68%) manifested these signs, the etiology of the cardiac dysfunction could almost always be attributed to pathogenic mechanisms related to the underlying diseases rather than directly to DIC (Table IX-I).

In one case cardiac dysfunction was directly attributable to DIC. Atrial fibrillation developed in a patient with purpura fulminans associated with pericardial hemorrhage (without tamponade). The small vessels of the pericardium contained thrombi at autopsy (*see* history of Case 6, Chap. IV).

A second patient had a cardiopulmonary arrest immediately after curettage of the uterus for a retained third trimester abortus. It is postulated that necrotic tissue debris with tissue

TABLE IX-I
ETIOLOGY OF CARDIAC DYSFUNCTION ASSOCIATED WITH DIC

Etiology of Dysfunction[1]	*# Patients*
Atherosclerosis	8
Volume overload	4
Myocarditis, septic endocarditis	4
Aortic vessel disease (dissection, coarctation)	3
Marantic endocarditis	2
Infiltrative (leukemic, amyloid)	2
Severe hypoxemia	1
? Amniotic fluid embolism	1
Pericardial hemorrhage and thrombosis 2° DIC	1
Total	26

[1] Coronary heart disease (atherosclerosis) required autopsy confirmation, or past history of angina or myocardial infarction antedating onset of DIC; endo- or myocarditis required autopsy confirmation; volume overload required rapid multiple transfusions when edema, acute renal failure, cor pulmonale, or old hypertensive cardiovascular diseases were present; severe hypoxemia required a $pO_2 < 40$ mmHg attributable to primary pulmonary disease.

thromboplastin may have been introduced into the maternal vascular system, thereby implanting into many maternal organs, including the brain and heart (105, 158). The consequence was DIC, local fibrin deposition, and probably the various observed forms of organ dysfunction (*see* history of Case 30, Chap. VI).

PULMONARY DYSFUNCTION

Many patients (78%) had clinical evidence of pulmonary dysfunction manifested by: dyspnea, hypoxemia, ($pO_2 < 80$ mm Hg on $FiO_2 > 50\%$), requirement for artificial ventilation, pulmonary congestion or acute chest X-ray abnormality suggestive of edema or hemorrhage (*see* Table IV-V).

Although the dysfunction in most of these thirty-three patients could be attributed to anatomic causes other than DIC (Table IX-II), in at least six patients the symptoms appeared causally related to pulmonary hemorrhage and DIC (175).

A synopsis of the manifestations of the syndrome of pulmonary hemorrhage and DIC is presented in Table IX-III. Clinically the syndrome was heralded by hemoptysis, dyspnea

TABLE IX-II
ETIOLOGY OF PULMONARY DYSFUNCTION ASSOCIATED WITH DIC

Etiology of Dysfunction[1]	*# Patients*
Pulmonary infection	11 (3 with hemorrhage)
Cardiac decompensation	9 (2 with hemorrhage)
Pulmonary hemorrhage and edema 2° DIC	6 (2 prostatic carcinoma, 4 acute leukemia)
Pleural effusion	2 (1 tumor, 1 cirrhosis)
Unexplained hypoxemia	2
Leukemic infiltrate with hemorrhage	1
Pulmonary emboli, recurrent	1
Total	32

[1] Pulmonary infection required extensive involvement; cardiac decompensation required pulmonary congestion with documented severe myocardial, aortic vessel disease, or acute volume overload; pulmonary hemorrhage required autopsy confirmation or the combination of hemoptysis and X-ray signs of a diffuse infiltrate.

or chest pain. Physical examination revealed rales, wheezing, marked tachypnea, and occasionally pleural friction rubs. Gallop heart sounds were rarely encountered, the blood pressure was stable, and the central venous pressure was not elevated. The chest X-ray commonly showed the pattern of a diffuse intra-alveolar infiltrate. Serial coagulation tests preceding and during the syndrome disclosed the changes expected during DIC, namely a falling hematocrit (from 41 to 29%), platelet count (from 154,000 to 24,000/ul), fibrinogen level (from 393 to 113 mg/dl), prolongation of the prothrombin time (from 13 to 18 sec), and elevated titers of FDP (1:74) (average values).

Autopsy revealed extensive pulmonary edema and hemorrhage; there was no anatomic evidence of cardiac or other pulmonary disease, including neoplastic infiltrates in the lung. Sample case histories are presented below, while the case histories of other patients with the syndrome are presented elsewhere (*see* history of Case 24, Chap. IV and Case 12, Chap. IX.) (80, Case 2 of Polliack [163] reviewed in 175).

CASE 27—ACUTE MYELOMONOCYTIC LEUKEMIA AND PULMONARY HEMORRHAGE: A 55-year-old white woman entered with easy bruising for three days. On admission the temperature was 101°. Ecchymoses dotted the shoulder and ankles. Bilateral basilar rales were audible and the spleen was enlarged. The hematocrit was 25%, WBC 19,700 with 87% myelomonocytic blast forms, 2% bands, and

TABLE IX-III

PULMONARY HEMORRHAGE SYNDROME

Case	Hemop-tysis	Dyspnea	Chest pain	Rales wheeze	Pleural friction rub	X-ray	Respiration (rate/min)	Blood pressure	Lung weight	Pulmonary Hemorrhage Causing death
12		+				"edema"	20→60	S→60 D→40	1300g	Yes
16	+	+	+	+	+	ND	20→30	Stable	1200g	Yes
21				+		ND	20→28	Stable	2000g	No
24	+		+	+		Diffuse	24→32	Stable	Alive	
27	+	+	+	+	+	Butterfly pattern	20→40	Stable	ND	Yes
29	+					Diffuse	20→25	S→60 D→40	ND	Yes

10% lymphocytes. The PT was normal, platelets 23,000/ul, and fibrinogen 480 gm/dl. The bone marrow contained 90% blasts, decreased megakaryocytes, and numerous megaloblasts. An initial chest X-ray disclosed an infiltrate in the right lower lobe.

Transfusions, penicillin, and 6-mercaptopurine were given. On the third day, the temperature rose to 104°F. An X-ray of the chest disclosed an enlarging right lower lobe infiltrate; since pneumonia was suspected, cephalothin was begun. The PT was normal, platelets 11,000/ul, and fibrinogen 552 mg/dl. The fever persisted. During the next several days, the infiltrate enlarged to involve predominantly the right middle lobe; the respiratory rate rose from 20 to 40, and the patient was obviously worse. On the seventh day splenic tenderness and diffuse pulmonary rales appeared.

X-rays of the chest showed extensive bilateral butterfly infiltrates. Marked respiratory distress occurred together with hemoptysis and right lateral pleuritic pain. During an eight hour period, pain was localized to an area where a friction rub was heard. Examination of the bloody sputum revealed no organisms. A two day trial of chloramphenicol and erythromycin was given. On the eleventh day high dose prednisolone therapy was begun (200 mg/day IV). Two days later, petechiae appeared on the trunk, purpura at pressure points, and venipuncture sites and the hemoptysis increased greatly.

The pulmonary symptoms increased; the respiratory rate was 40. Rare helmet cells were observed in peripheral smears of blood. Over the next four days the hematocrit fell (despite transfusions) from 31% to 24%, the PT rose to 17 sec, and fibrinogen fell from 430 to 96 mg/dl. The platelets were 7000/ul. Heparin (6000 U every 4 hr) was begun. Over two days the PT fell to 14 sec, while the fibrinogen rose to 288 mg/dl. The respiratory distress increased and she died one day later. Autopsy was not performed.

Comment: This case is an example of the pulmonary hemorrhage syndrome complicating acute leukemia.

CASE 16 (FIG. IX-1)—PROMYELOCYTIC LEUKEMIA, RECURRENT DIC AND PULMONARY HEMORRHAGE: A 50-year-old man entered with spontaneous ecchymoses, epistaxis, gross hematuria, and oral mucosal hemorrhage. The hematocrit was 34%, WBC 4100 with 70% promyelocytes. The tests of hemostasis were mildly abnormal (Fig. IX-1). A bone marrow was hypercellular with 90% promyelocytes. Erythroid elements and megakaryocytes were markedly decreased. Prednisone and 6-mercaptopurine were administered. The hematuria persisted whereas the epistaxis abated. On the sixth hospital day the hematocrit fell to 26%. Despite administration of 3 units of fresh whole blood and 10 units of platelet concentrates, the tests of clotting function became more abnormal during the next three days. However, factors II, V, and VII-X were 175%, 89% and 100% of normal.

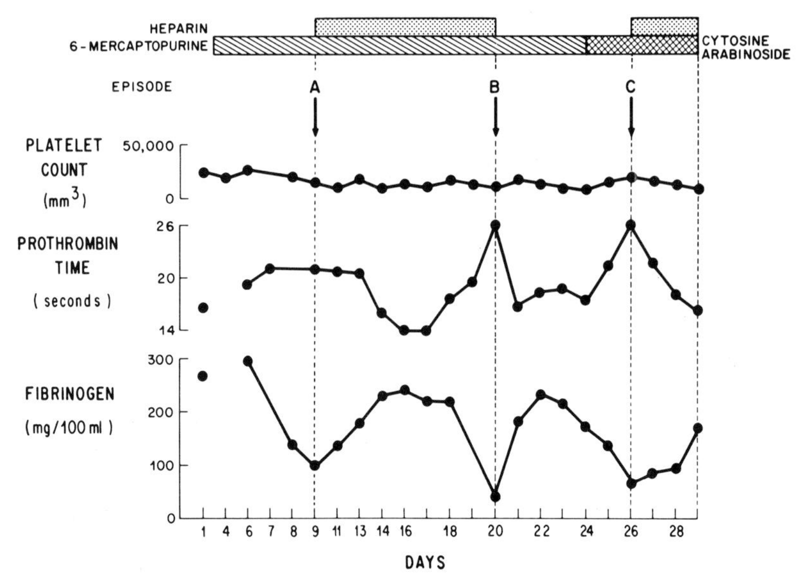

Figure IX–1. Case 16.

Heparin (6000 U every 4 hr) was started. No new bleeding developed and by the sixteenth hospital day the coagulation tests returned towards normal. The hematocrit was 30–35% and WBC 800 with 10% promyelocytes, 68% lymphocytes. A bone marrow examination was unchanged. Two days later a large axillary hematoma and recurrent epistaxis appeared. The hematocrit fell to 16%, and the tests of clotting function became abnormal. The hematomas continued to enlarge. Eight units of fresh blood were given and the heparin was stopped.

On the twenty-fourth day cystosine arabinoside was substituted for 6-mercaptopurine. Two days later klebsiella septicemia developed associated with hematoma formation, rise in PT, and fall in fibrinogen level. Severe chest pain, pleural rubs, wheezing, tachypnea and hemoptysis appeared. The respiratory rate rose from 20 to 30 and the pulse from 90 to 120; the blood pressure remained stable. Shortly thereafter wheezes were heard throughout the entire right chest while breath sounds diminished. One hour later both the wheezing and the chest pain were more prominent. Four hours later death occurred.

Autopsy disclosed acute promyelocytic leukemia involving bone marrow, spleen, and kidney. The lung contained extensive hemorrhage, but no tumor or bronchopneumonia. Other findings included hematomas and purpura involving the right shoulder, back, arms, adrenal pelves, and left ureter and fibrin thrombi in skin and renal glomeruli.

Comment: This case illustrates the pulmonary hemorrhage syndrome as a cause of death. The patient had three episodes of DIC. At least one and possibly two of the episodes were associated temporally with chemotherapy.

PATIENT 21—PROMYELOCYTIC LEUKEMIA, PULMONARY AND CENTRAL NERVOUS SYSTEM HEMORRHAGE: A 33-year-old man entered for epistaxis and progressive fatigue of six weeks' duration. On admission numerous ecchymoses covered the thorax and extremities. Fundal hemorrhages, infected bleeding gingiva, bleeding from venipuncture sites, melena, and splenomegaly were observed. The hematocrit was 15%, WBC 11,450 with 85% promyelocytes. The PT was 25 sec, platelets 19,000/ul, fibrinogen 160 mg/dl, Fi 1:80, ELT immediate. The bone marrow was packed with 20% myeloblasts and 75% promyelocytes. Heparin (7250 U every 4 hr), allopurinol, and four units of fresh whole blood were given. One day later cytosine arabinoside, 6-mercaptopurine, penicillin, and EACA (4 gm IV priming dose, then 1 gm hourly) were added. During the next three days the bleeding subsided and the hematocrit rose to 29%.

On the fifth day petechiae erupted on the skin and mucosal membranes, a large antecubital hematoma developed at the site of an intravenous cannula, the retinal hemorrhages enlarged and palpable ecchymoses appeared over the abdominal wall. The WBC was 41,000 with 91% promyelocytes, fibrinogen 100 mg/dl, platelets 7000/ul, and PT 25 sec. Tachypnea, rales, new fundal hemorrhage and signs of decerebration appeared and the patient suddenly died.

Autopsy showed acute promyelocytic leukemia involving the spleen, liver, kidney and lymph nodes. Fibrin thrombi were present in renal glomerular capillaries. The lungs were hemorrhagic but showed neither leukemic infiltrates nor bronchopneumonia. Examination of the brain was not permitted.

Comment: Pulmonary and central nervous system hemorrhage developed in association with a generalized worsening of a fulminant hemorrhagic diathesis.

MONKEY #139—PULMONARY HEMORRHAGE SYNDROME AND RENAL FAILURE FOLLOWING THE EXPERIMENTAL INDUCTION OF DIC: A healthy female *Macaca irus* monkey was challenged by intravenous infusion of 150 hemolytic units of IgG derived from the plasma of a donor alloimmunized with red cells.* Within 30 minutes of infusion, the respiratory rate rose from 25 to 60 and severe respiratory distress was evident. The hematocrit fell from 38 to 18% while initially the blood pressure remained stable. The platelet count fell from 364,000 to 96,000/ul, fibrinogen from 303 to 103 mg/dl, factor V from 96% to 42%, factor VII from 111% to 40%, factor

* A hemolytic unit is defined as the amount of purified hemolytic IgG necessary to produce 50% hemolysis in an in vitro test system containing 3% red cells in saline and complement (107).

VIII from 240% to 59%, factor IX from 104% to 23%, factor X from 95% to 30%, factor XI from 200% to 93% and factor XII from 208% to 80%. The urine volume fell from 7.0 ml/min to 1.0 ml at 5 minutes and to 0.5 ml at 60 minutes, while the specific gravity rose from 1.033 to 1.045 and the urine hemoglobin rose from 0.66 mg to over 2000 mg/dl. The plasma hemoglobin rose from a preinfusion value of 11 mg/dl (normal 19 ± 11 mg/dl) to over 1000 mg/dl.

Shortly before the animal died one hour after infusion, the respiratory distress was severe and bloody nasal froth was observed. A continuous electrocardiogram disclosed the appearance of giant P waves, followed by asystole.

Autopsy revealed numerous pulmonary hemorrhages (Fig. IX-2). Microscopically, multiple fibrin thrombi were present in renal glomeruli and in small arterial and venous vessels in the lungs (Fig. X-6).

Comment: This case illustrates that the pulmonary hemorrhage syndrome can be produced in the absence of both tumor and septicemia.

The pulmonary hemorrhage syndrome is not an infrequent complication of DIC occurring in 10 to 20 percent of patients with hemorrhagic manifestations. It should be consid-

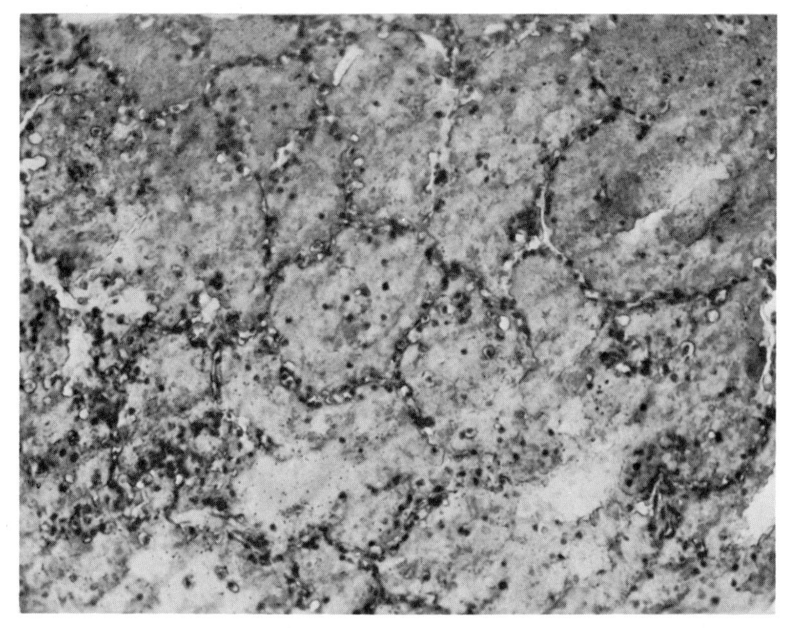

Figure IX–2. Pulmonary hemorrhage in a monkey in which DIC was experimentally produced. (Hematoxylin and eosin stain, × 190).

ered when signs of respiratory distress, hemoptysis, and pleuritic chest pain are apparent or when unexplained infiltrates develop in the chest X-ray. Although we have identified the syndrome in the settings of acute leukemia and prostatic carcinoma, pulmonary hemorrhage of rather severe degree was also documented at autopsy in association with bacterial pneumonias, which in contrast was usually of minimal degree. McGovern (113) has reported similar findings; pulmonary hemorrhage frequently occurred with gram negative septicemia (67% of 49 patients).

The routine differential diagnosis of respiratory distress in patients with DIC should include: pulmonary edema secondary to volume overload or cardiac failure, bronchopneumonia, pulmonary emboli, oxygen toxicity, hemothorax, transfusion reactions, aspiration or pulmonary involvement with neoplastic process. Although systematic trials of therapy have not been conducted, it appears that the pulmonary hemorrhage will only be controlled with control of DIC and the underlying disease precipitating it. Since pulmonary hemorrhage is often fatal, recognition and prompt institution of therapy are important.

An animal model suggests that the pulmonary hemorrhage syndrome is secondary to the DIC rather than to neoplasia or other diseases which trigger DIC (175), and should permit a systematic study of various therapeutic modalities. Intravenous administration of anti-red cell antibodies causes massive rapid intravascular hemolysis in monkeys. Severe DIC is readily and reproducibly initiated (109). Associated with the DIC the animals show severe dyspnea, tachypnea, experience hemoptysis and have giant P waves on electrocardiogram. At necropsy pulmonary hemorrhage (Fig. IX-2) and in some cases multiple fibrin thrombi in arterioles and venules (Fig. X-6) are found (108,175).

Some patients with DIC have transient hypoxemia that is unexplained and without coincident radiographic manifestations (*see* history of Case 31, Chap. IV). The hypoxemia disappears as the episode of DIC resolves. Possibly the hypoxemia is secondary to transient involvement of pulmonary vasculature with fibrin thrombi and the subsequent resolution by fibrinolysis.

RENAL DYSFUNCTION

Many patients (67%) have clinical evidence of renal dysfunction manifested by: oliguria (less than 500 ml of urine output/day), serum creatinine greater than 2.0 mg/dl, blood urea nitrogen greater than 40 mg/dl, or hematuria (*see* Table IV-V). With rare exceptions the etiology of the renal dysfunction could be attributed to pathogenic mechanisms related to the underlying diseases rather than directly to DIC (Table IX-IV). Hypovolemia, low cardiac output (cardiogenic shock syndrome), acute tubular necrosis, or chronic renal disease with an acute insult (infection, obstruction or toxic drugs) accounted for the majority of patients with renal dysfunction.

Acute tubular necrosis occurred in association with DIC rather frequently. Usually this was related to a known cause of hypotension developing prior to DIC. A few patients had ATN develop concurrently with DIC and were subsequently found to have glomerular fibrin thrombi at necropsy (*see* history of Case 12 below).

TABLE IX-IV
ETIOLOGY OF RENAL DYSFUNCTION
ASSOCIATED WITH DIC

Etiology of Dysfunction[1]	*# Patients*
Acute tubular necrosis syndrome	8
prior to DIC (2)	
concurrent with DIC	
related to hypotension that precipitated DIC (4)	
probably related to DIC (2)	
Chronic renal disease with acute insult	7
Pre-renal, non-vascular	5
Hematuria without oliguria or azotemia	4
2° to leukemic infiltrate, carcinoma, Foley catheter	
Aspergillus pyelonephritis	2
Meningococcemia, fulminant with glomerular fibrin thrombi	2
Renal infarct, emboli	1
Unexplained	1
Total	30

[1] Acute tubular necrosis (ATN) required oliguria, azotemia, and appropriate urine electrolytes (urine sodium > 20 mEq/L, urine osmolarity < 400 mosm/L); chronic renal disease required prior evaluation or histological documentation, and an acute documented insult such as infection, obstruction, or toxin (e.g., large doses of kanamycin or colistin), or prolonged hypotension; pre-renal etiology represented severe hypovolemia, or low cardiac output resulting in cardiogenic shock syndrome with a documented cardiac lesion.

CASE 12—PROSTATIC CARCINOMA, ACUTE TUBULAR NECROSIS AND PULMONARY HEMORRHAGE: Nine years previously a radical prostatectomy disclosed adenocarcinoma and six years later skeletal metastases developed. On admission X-rays showed radiodense nodules throughout the skeleton. The hematocrit was 20% but there was no sign of bleeding. The PT was 13 sec and platelets were normal on blood smear examination. Urinalysis, renal and liver function were normal.

On the fifth day testosterone (100 mg/day) and ^{32}P (2 mCi IV) were given. Within one day profound epistaxis, mucosal bleeding, hematuria, and venipuncture site bleeding appeared. The platelets were 29,000/ul, PT 23 sec, fibrinogen 60 mg/dl, Fi test 1:160, and clotting time 2 hours. The kallikrein system was normal (Table VIII-III). Vitamin K, heparin (6250 U every 4 hr), EACA (1 gm IV hr), fresh frozen plasma, fresh whole blood, and 6 gm of fibrinogen were administered. On the next day the temperature rose to 105° F and he became hypotensive, dyspneic, and severely oliguric. Hemoptysis, hematemesis, melena and increased wound bleeding occurred and *E. coli* was cultured from the blood. The BUN was 66 mg and creatinine 3.9 mg/dl, and urinalysis showed gross hematuria without casts. Subsequently the fibrinogen rose to 174 mg/dl, PT fell to 18 sec, platelets rose to 43,000/ul and the bleeding subsided, but he remained profoundly hypotensive, and died on the ninth day.

Autopsy revealed adenocarcinoma of the prostate with widespread metastases, pulmonary hemorrhage and edema (but without pulmonary tumor). Bilateral renal pelvic hemorrhage without obstruction was present. There was acute tubular necrosis but only rare fibrin thrombi in the renal glomerular capillaries.

Comment: The temporal relation between the administration of chemotherapeutic agents and the onset of DIC was striking. One day after the DIC appeared, the patient developed septicemia with severe hypotension, more bleeding, signs of the pulmonary hemorrhage syndrome, and acute renal failure. Pathophysiologically the acute tubular necrosis could have been secondary to the bout of hypotension or to deposition of fibrin thrombi after EACA and fibrinogen therapy.

Occasionally transient hematuria and mild azotemia occur simultaneously with DIC when no other explanations are present, (*see* history of Case 31, Chap. IV). The changes in renal function are probably related to DIC since they occur characteristically in monkeys when DIC is experimentally produced (107,108). Although the pathophysiologic mechanism is unknown, Kincaid-Smith *et al.* (92) have shown that a platelet-fibrin thrombus is implicated.

A well documented example of renal dysfunction induced by DIC is the acute local (intrarenal) DIC that is associated with acute homograft rejection of the transplanted kidney (27,28). Although these patients demonstrate no evidence of systemic intravascular coagulation, fibrin degradation products and decreased coagulation factors are found in renal vein effluent.

NERVOUS SYSTEM DYSFUNCTION

Many patients had clinical evidence of nervous system dysfunction manifested by: coma, delirium, seizures, stroke syndrome, Babinski responses, clonus, cranial nerve signs, paraplegia, or sensory loss (see Table IV-V). Although twenty-nine patients (65%) manifested these signs, most had severe metabolic devects, CNS infections or emboli as the etiology of the dysfunction. However, several patients had lesions that appeared to be directly related to DIC (Cases 4, 15 17, 30) (Table IX-V). Spontaneous intracerebral bleeding occurred in one patient (*see* history of Case 4, Chap. XIII) while in

TABLE IX-V

ETIOLOGY OF NEUROLOGIC DYSFUNCTION ASSOCIATED WITH DIC

Etiology of Dysfunction[1]	*# Patients*
Severe metabolic	14
CNS infection	6
Embolic, heart valve	2
Leukemic infiltrate	1
CNS bleeding	4
associated with leukemic infiltrate (2)	
spontaneous (1)	
? heparin complication (1)	
CNS thrombosis	2
EACA therapy alone (1)	
? amniotic fluid emboli,	
Total	29

[1] Severe metabolic classification represented combination of three of the following simultaneously: fever > 105 F, hypoxia, hypotension, acidosis, azotemia, severe respiratory acidosis ($pCO_2 > 100$ mmHg), or hepatic encephalopathy. CNS hemorrhage required documentation by examination of cerebral spinal fluid (CSF) or necropsy; CNS thrombosis required autopsy documentation or stroke syndrome with no blood in the CSF; CNS infection required bacteriological or histological confirmation. Figures in parentheses represent numbers of patients in the individual groups.

two patients the hemorrhage or thrombosis occurred in the spinal cord (*see* histories of Case 17, Chap. XI and Case 15, Chap. XI). The last patient had a brainstem and cortical stroke syndrome that developed immediately after uterine curettage for a retained abortus.

The development of neurologic signs or symptoms in a patient with DIC is ominous. A large fraction of these patients subsequently died. Thus coma, delirium, focal neurologic signs and stroke syndromes should be carefully and fully evaluated. Besides documentation of the extent and location of the neurologic defect, examination should include determination of arterial pH, pO_2, pCO_2, liver function tests, cerebrospinal fluid examination and culture, and careful cardiac auscultation to detect possible embolic sources. The possibility of occult CNS meningeal infection or brain abscess with opportunistic organisms should be considered. In patients with leukemia the possibility of CNS leukemia should be strongly considered even if blood is present in the CSF.

Despite the frequent association of DIC with meningococcal meningitis and meningococcemia, there are infrequently severe CNS symptoms in these conditions.

Increased bleeding secondary to heparin therapy must be carefully considered although in our experience other factors usually precipitated the hemorrhage (*see* history of Case 17, Chap. XI). Guidelines for evaluation of increased bleeding during heparin therapy are given in Chapter XI.

Summary

Most patients with DIC have signs and symptoms of severe dysfunction of major organ systems (cardiac, pulmonary, renal or central nervous system). In the majority of these patients, factors other than DIC underlie their organ system dysfunction.

Cardiac dysfunction is usually related to atherosclerotic coronary artery disease, infection, or volume overload. Pulmonary dysfunction is often related to infection or cardiac decompensation. Renal dysfunction is related to hypovolemia, diminished cardiac function and hypotension induced acute tubular necrosis, sepsis or chronic renal disease. Nervous system dysfunction is related primarily to metabolic defects (fever, hypoxia, hypotension, acidosis, liver failure) and to infection.

The syndrome of pulmonary hemorrhage and edema appears to be related causally to DIC. It carries an ominous prognosis.

CHAPTER X

PATHOLOGY

THE AUTOPSY IS INVALUABLE IN understanding the response of the diseased host to underlying diseases as well as to ongoing DIC. Not only does the autopsy help identify the multiple (and often unsuspected) disease processes present in each patient, but it can aid in determining the relative importance of each and the effect that therapy may have had in ameliorating the impact of each. The autopsy also helps to assign the cause of clinical signs and symptoms to specific disease entities.

Elsewhere, the types and extent of the multiple disease processes other than DIC are described in detail (*see* Chap. III, IX, XI, XII, and individual case histories). This chapter deals specifically with the pathological features related to DIC, in particular its manifestations in the skin and major blood vessels, and the significance of the fibrin thrombus.

One section correlates clinical, coagulation, autopsy findings and attempts to assign to each a relative importance in causing death.

Lastly a problem-oriented guide is presented by which an autopsy might be performed when DIC is suspected.

AUTOPSY FINDINGS

The spectrum of pathological findings in DIC includes fibrin thrombi, major vessel thrombosis, small vessel thrombosis, hemorrhage, and their complications. Tables X-I and X-II present postmortem examination data for our patients. The pathological hallmark of DIC is the fibrin thrombus. With hematoxylin and eosin stained tissue sections, the fibrin thrombus is a dense mass made up of tightly woven homogeneous eosinophilic strands. The thrombus is rarely adherent to the vascular wall and usually no inflammatory

TABLE X-I
AUTOPSY DATA

Case	*Location of Thrombi*	*Miscellaneous Data*
4	Liver	Lung hyaline membranes; cerebral bleeding spontaneous
5	Lung, kidney, testis	Pulmonary and cerebral hemorrhages with leukemic infiltrates
6	Adrenal, colon, lung, skin, spleen, testis, vasa vasorum of aorta	Thrombosis, dorsal vein penis; cardiac dysfunction 2° disseminated intravascular coagulation
8	Colon, heart, kidney, spleen, testis	Subclavian vein thrombosis and pulmonary emboli 2° catheter; marantic endocarditis
12	Kidney	Pulmonary hemorrhage, no carcinoma infiltrate; acute tubular necrosis ? 2° disseminated intravascular coagulation
15	Anterior median spinal artery	Spinal cord infarct 2° to epsilon-aminocaproic acid therapy; mural thrombus in aortic aneurysm
16	Kidney, skin	Pulmonary hemorrhage without leukemic infiltrate; cerebral bleeding with leukemic infiltrate
18	No thrombi	——
19	Adrenal, skin	Mural thrombus in aneurysm
20	Choroid plexus, heart, kidney, lung, skin	Adrenal hemorrhage
21	Kidney	Pulmonary hemorrhage without and cerebral bleeding with leukemic infiltrate
22	Adrenal, colon, kidney	Large vessel thrombosis ? 2° catheter
28	Heart, kidney, pancreas, skin	Aspergillus hyphae in major vessels of kidney, brain, thyroid
32	Kidney	Renal artery aneurysm with renal infarct; lung emboli and hyaline membranes
33	Adrenal, colon, kidney, seminal vesicles, skin, spleen, testis, muscle	Multiple thrombosed vessels and pulmonary emboli 2° catheters; lung hyaline membranes
35	Kidney	Bleeding duodenal ulcer
38	Choroid plexus, kidney, prostate, skin, testis	Superior vena cava mural thrombus and pulmonary emboli 2° catheter; left ventricular mural thrombus
39	Pancreas, skin	
40	Lung	Marantic endocarditis
42	Kidney, liver, lung, pituitary, skin, testis	Adrenal hemorrhage
43	Kidney, skin	Lung hyaline membranes; multiple thrombosed vessels 2° catheters
45	Kidney	Aspergillus hyphae in major vessels of kidney, brain

(Robboy, Colman and Minna: *Hum Path*, 3:327, 1972)

TABLE X-II
LOCATION OF FIBRIN THROMBI IN 22 AUTOPSIES AND
7 SKIN BIOPSIES

	Number		Frequency (%)
Thrombi, any location	26/29		90
Kidney	15/22		68
Skin	15/29		52
Lung	11/22		50
Thrombi		5	
Pulmonary emboli		4	
Hyaline (fibrin) membranes		3	
Pulmonary hemorrhage syndrome		4	
Testis	6/13		46
Major Blood vessels (excluding aorta)	9/22		41
Vein			
Central venous pressure catheter		5	
Cardiac electrode		1	
Artery			
Catheter		2	
Puncture		1	
Aspergillus		2	
Miscellaneous		2	
Heart	6/22		27
Thrombi		3	
Marantic endocarditis		2	
Mural thrombus		2	
Adrenal	6/22		27
Thrombi		4	
Diffuse hemorrhage		2	
Central nervous system	5/22		23
Spleen	3/22		14
Aorta	3/22		14
Aneurysm with thrombus		2	
Vasa vasorum		1	
Thyroid	2/22		9
Liver	2/22		9
Pancreas	2/22		9
Other organs	2/22		9

(Robboy, Colman and Minna: *Hum Path*, 3:327, 1972)

reaction is invoked. We were able to find fibrin thrombi in nearly all the patients. The number of organs containing thrombi usually varied from one to eight while the maximal number of organs involved in any case was thirteen (Case 33).

Fibrin thrombi are observed more frequently in the kidney (68%) than in any other organ. This fact that may be explained by the pathogenesis of the thrombi. McKay (116) has suggested that most thrombi form in the systemic circulation as fibrin aggregates and that by a sieving effect they are eventually caught in smaller vessels. Because of its rich microvasculature and high blood flow the kidney thus acts as an excellent sieve. As the fibrin aggregates are forced into yet smaller vessels, the red cells are squeezed out and the characteristic tight fibrin thrombus is formed. An example of this is shown in Figure X-1 where the clot present in the distal afferent arteriole (hilus of glomerulus) is seen to be composed of loose strands of fibrin, whereas in the glomerular capillaries it is tightly woven fibrin. In contrast, fetuses have a large blood flow from the placenta through the liver, and in the stillborn

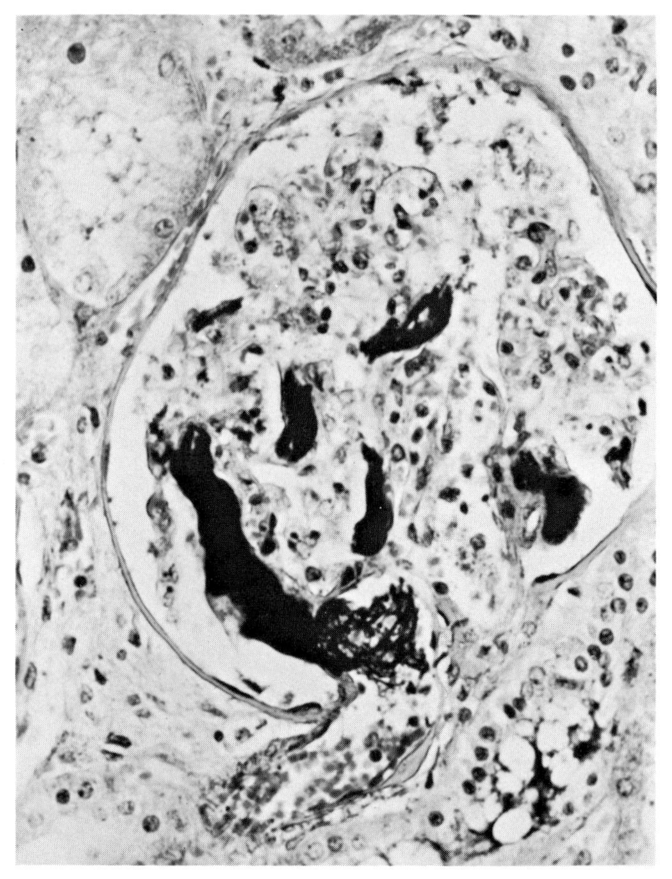

Figure X–1. Multiple fibrin thrombi in glomerulus. The fibrin in the terminal afferent arteriole (hilus of glomerulus) is loose and in strands, whereas it is compact in the capillaries. Case 32. (Phosphotungstic acid-hematoxylin stain, × 380.) (Robboy, Colman, Minna: *Hum Pathol, 3*:327, 1972.)

infant the liver is the organ most commonly affected by the thrombi (13).

Fibrin thrombi usually involve 2 to 10 percent of glomeruli. In many cases the thrombi are easily identified (Fig. X-1) but not uncommonly only a rare thrombus is detected after multiple blocks of tissue are sampled (Fig. X-2,3). The number of thrombi does not correlate with the duration nor severity of DIC nor with the magnitude of the fibrinolytic response measured by FDP titer, TT or ELT. Renal thrombi did not adhere to the glomerular basement membranes or show histologic evidence of organization. Although renal cortical necrosis (Shwartzman phenomenon) may occur in DIC (116) this phenomenon was not seen in any of our patients.

Fibrin thrombi can be demonstrated in the adrenal gland, central nervous system, heart, lung and testis in about one-fourth to one-half the cases. The thrombi are present in small

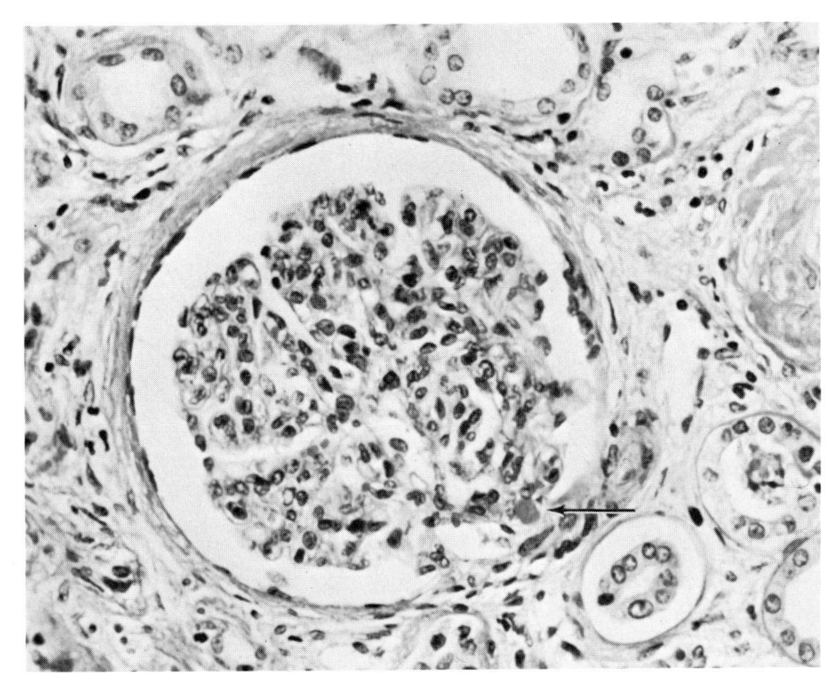

Figure X–2. Single fibrin thrombus (arrow) in glomerulus. Case 35. (Hematoxylin and eosin stain, × 360.) (*Ibid.*)

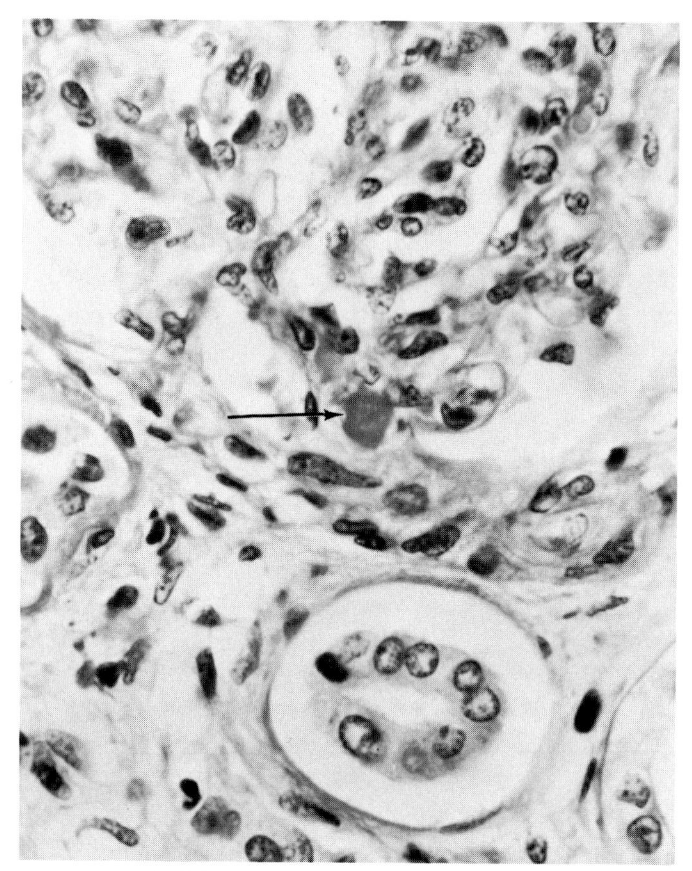

Figure X–3. Detail of fibrin thrombus in Figure X–2. (Hematoxylin and eosin stain, × 720.)

vessels, namely, the arterioles, capillaries, and venules, and rarely are numerous in any tissue section (Fig. X 4-7). On occasion multiple thrombi are closely packed in a small region, especially in the choroid plexus (Fig. X-8), and sometimes the presence of the thrombi can be suspected grossly by the finding of petechiae (Fig. X-9) or larger foci of hemorrhage (Fig. X-10). Usually the thrombi float freely within the vessel lumen, and only rarely are they adherent to vessel walls and superficially organized. (Fig. X-11).

PATHOLOGY OF THE SKIN

A variety of skin lesions (petechiae, purpura, purpura fulminans, gangrene, acral cyanosis, hemorrhagic bullae) regard-

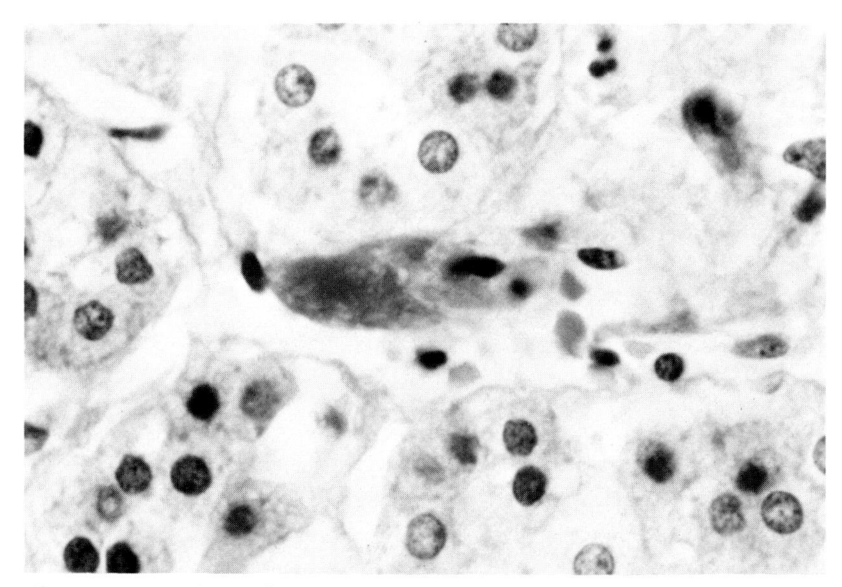

Figure X–4. Solitary fibrin thrombus in sinusoid of adrenal cortex. Case 6. (Hematoxylin and eosin stain, × 950.) (*Ibid.*)

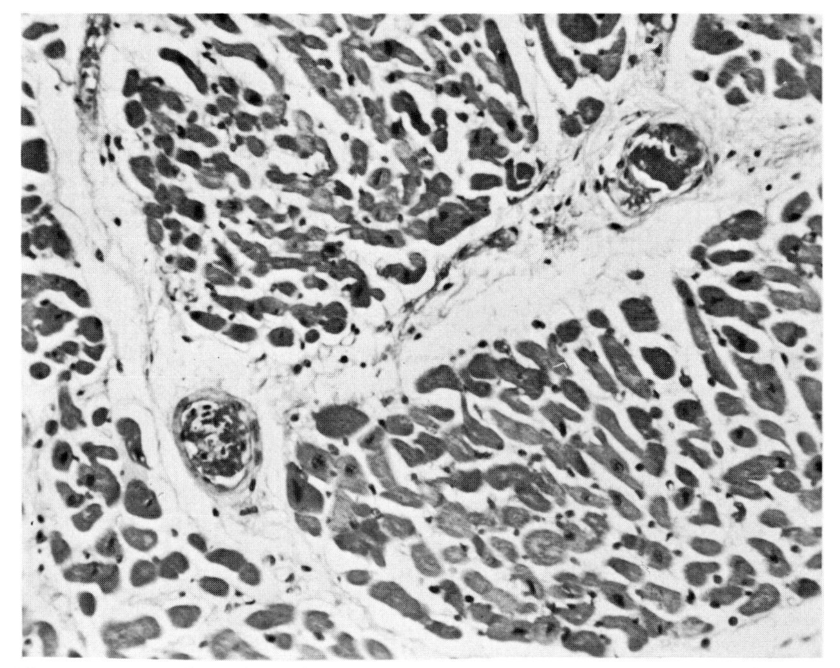

Figure X–5. Fibrin thrombi in cardiac vessels. Case 28. (Hematoxylin and eosin stain, × 210.) (*Ibid.*)

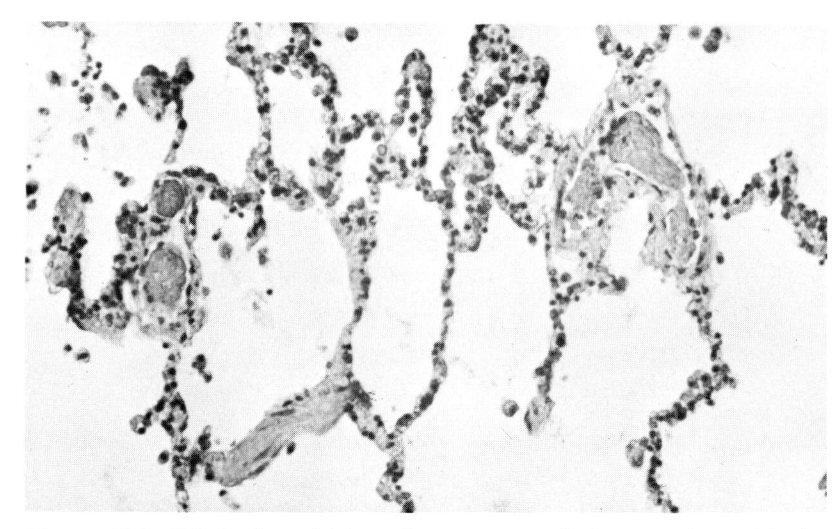

Figure X–6. Fibrin thrombi in pulmonary vessels in a monkey with the pulmonary hemorrhage syndrome. The DIC was experimentally produced. (Hematoxylin and eosin stain, × 260.)

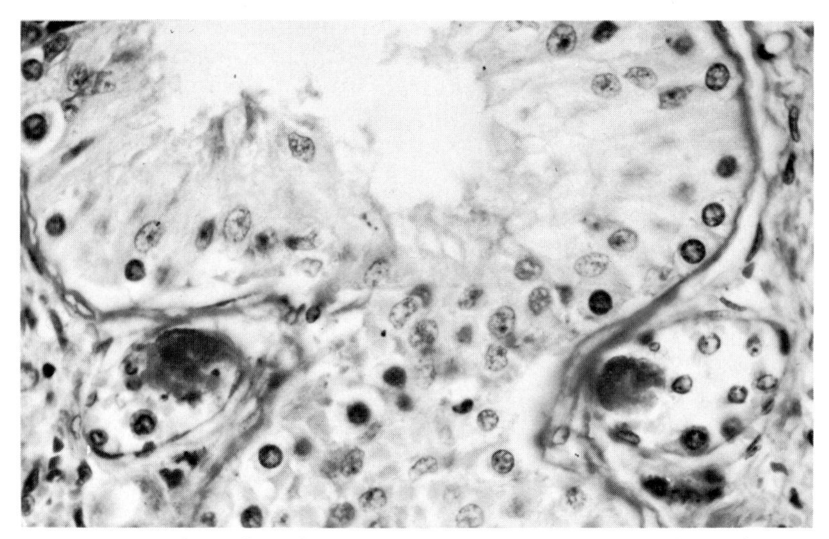

Figure X–7. Fibrin thrombi in testicle. Case 42. (Hematoxylin and eosin stain, × 485.)

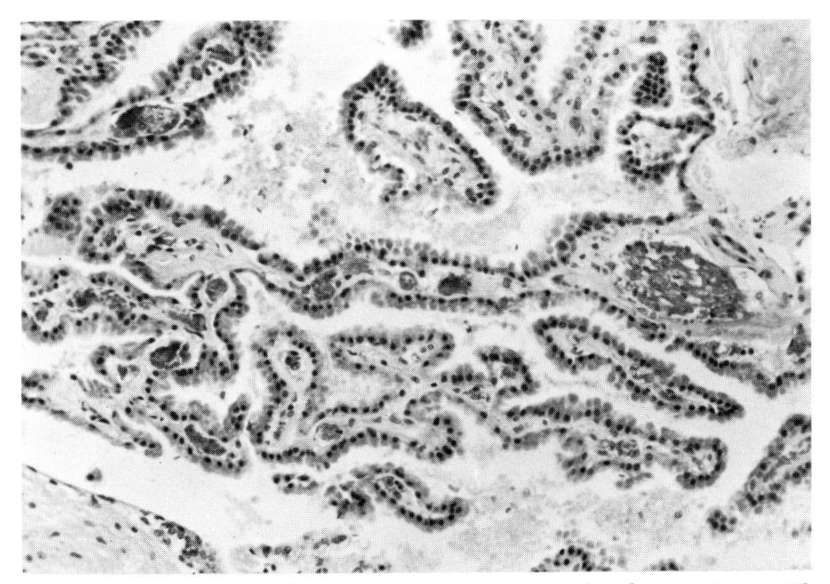

Figure X–8. Multiple fibrin thrombi in choroid plexus. Case 38. (Hematoxylin and eosin stain, × 170.) (*Ibid.*)

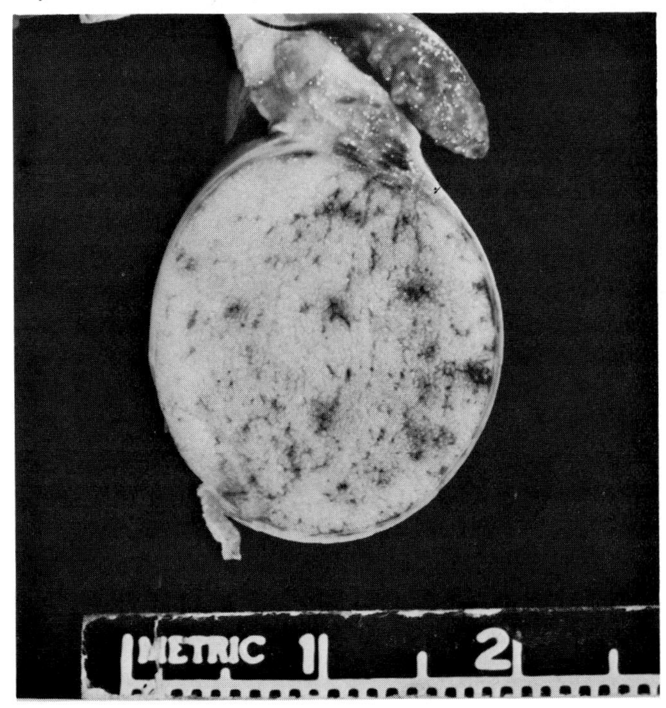

Figure X–9. Testicle petechiae. Microscopic examination revealed numerous fibrin thrombi. See Figure X–7. (*Ibid.*)

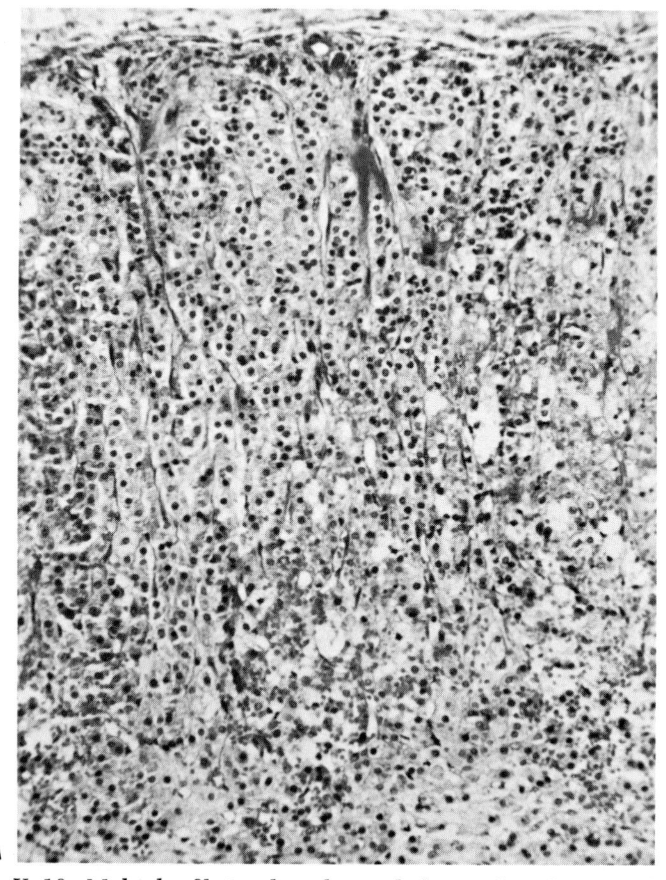

Figure X–10. Multiple fibrin thrombi occluding adrenal sinusoids. The cortical necrosis ranges in areas from minimal (A) to extensive (B). Case 22. (Hematoxylin and eosin stain, × 160 (A), 130 (B).) (*Ibid.*)

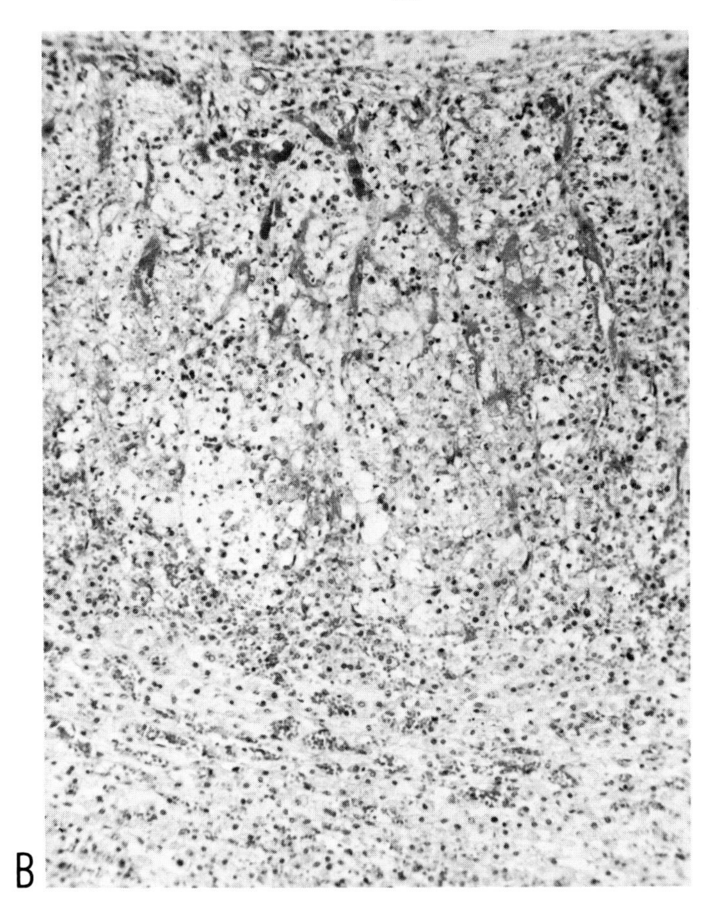
B

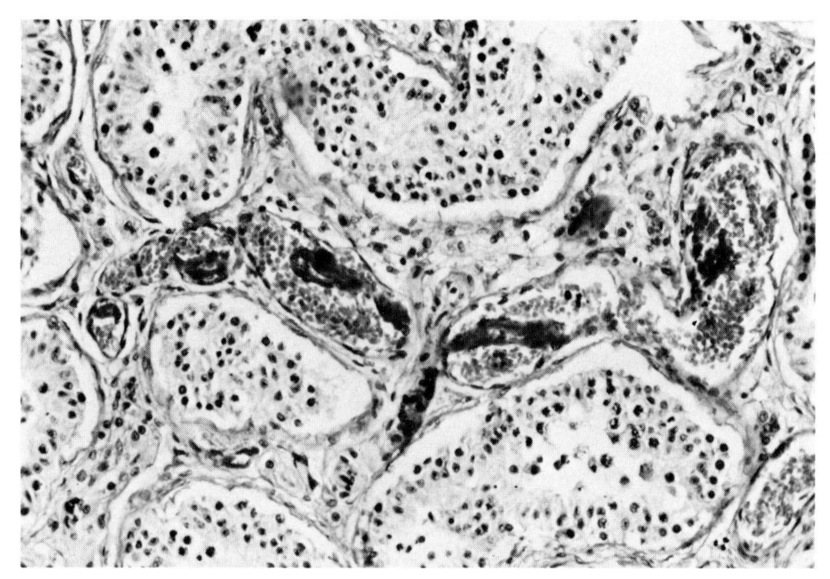

Figure X–11. Multiple fibrin thrombi in testicle, showing superficial organization, endothelialization and adherence to vessel wall. EACA was administered six days before death. Case 33. (Hematoxylin and eosin stain, × 170.) (*Ibid.*)

less of age will have fibrin thrombi. In lesions less than one day old, fibrin thrombi are present in the capillaries (Fig. X-12) and venules of the papillary dermis (Fig. X-13) and occasionally in the reticular dermis and subcutaneous tissue. Hemorrhage is present, but there is little or no epidermal necrosis and no inflammatory reaction (Fig. X-14).

Biopsies of older lesions (two to three days) reveals epidermal necrosis, formation of subepidermal bullae (Fig. X-15), extensive hemorrhage, and patchy necrosis of the eccrine glands, pilosebaceous apparatus, and papillary layer of the dermis (Fig. X-16). These manifestations probably reflect local ischemia, since they are accentuated whenever nearby blood vessels are thrombosed. Lesions that progress to gangrene or confluent ecchymoses (purpura fulminans-like picture) show extensive necrosis of the epidermis, dermis, and cutaneous appendages (Figs. X-17–19) and organizing thrombi of large vessels (Fig. X-20). Despite extensive necrosis, inflammatory responses are not observed.

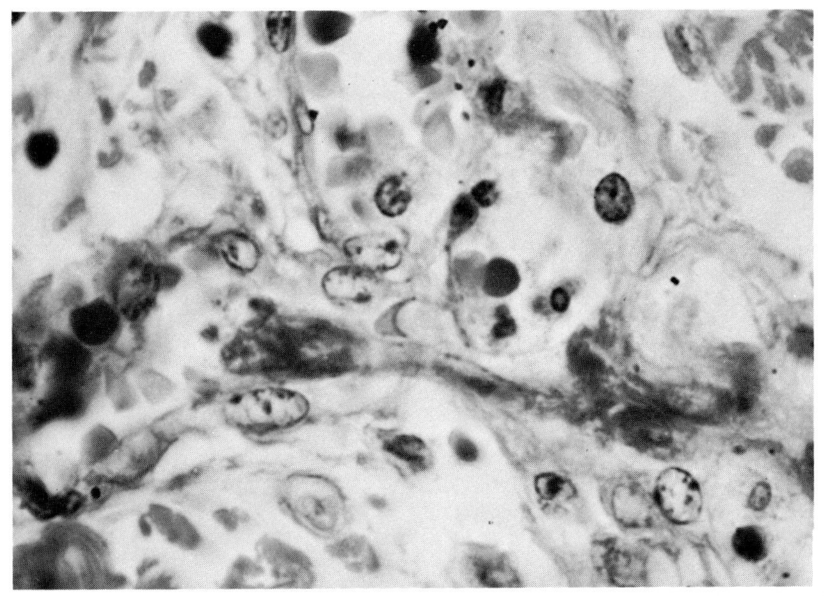

Figure X–12. Fibrin thrombus in a superficial vessel of the reticular dermis skin. The biopsy was obtained within several hours after the patient entered the hospital. There is no inflammatory reaction present. Case 20. (Hematoxylin and eosin stain, × 1180.)

Biopsy of skin lesions can be useful when the diagnosis of DIC is equivocal by coagulation test data. When skin biopsies were done in seven of our patients, five had evidence of fibrin thrombi. The subsequent clinical course, coagulation test changes, or autopsy material confirmed the diagnosis of DIC in all seven. One of these seven patients had gonococcemia and had the only biopsy specimen in this series in which an intense perivascular lymphocytic infiltrate was observed (Fig. X-21). The infiltrate is probably not due to DIC since we have found this type of infiltrate present in several other biopsy specimens of gonococcemia we have examined where there was no evidence of DIC (absence of thrombi and negative FDP titers).

Since petechiae and purpura are commonly associated with hematological diseases, their appearance in DIC usually leads to appropriate hematological evaluation. However, necrotic skin lesions, acral cyanosis and hemorrhagic bullae have previously been ascribed to vasculitis, embolic disease, allergic

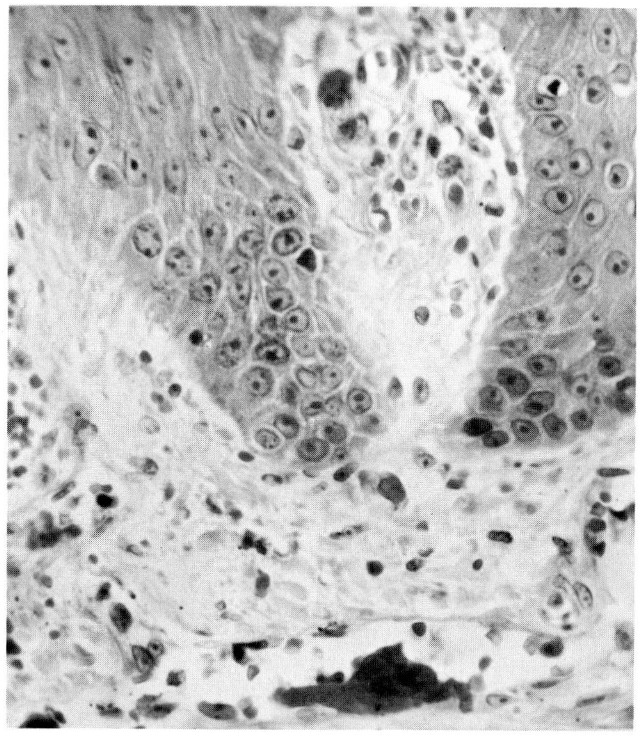

Figure X–13. Fibrin thrombus in a vessel of the papillary dermis of the skin. There is slight extravasation of red blood cells, but no inflammation. (Hematoxylin and eosin stain, × 720.)

eruptions or poor cardiovascular states and only recently has their association with DIC been noted (173).

Since the pathological hallmark of DIC is the fibrin thrombus, the vessel wall may occasionally exhibit necrosis, but is not inflamed. The epidermis is not affected, unless secondarily by ischemia. These findings make it possible to distinguish DIC from other lesions causing palpable purpura (septic emboli, allergic cutaneous vasculitis, systemic necrotizing angiitis), hemorrhagic bullae (erythema multiforme, and bullous pemphigoid), or acral cyanosis (Raynaud's phenomenon, chilblains, or acrocyanosis) (104,133,189).

It is important to remember that in any of the above conditions, especially allergic cutaneous vasculitis or subepidermal bullous disorders, septicemia or shock may intervene and

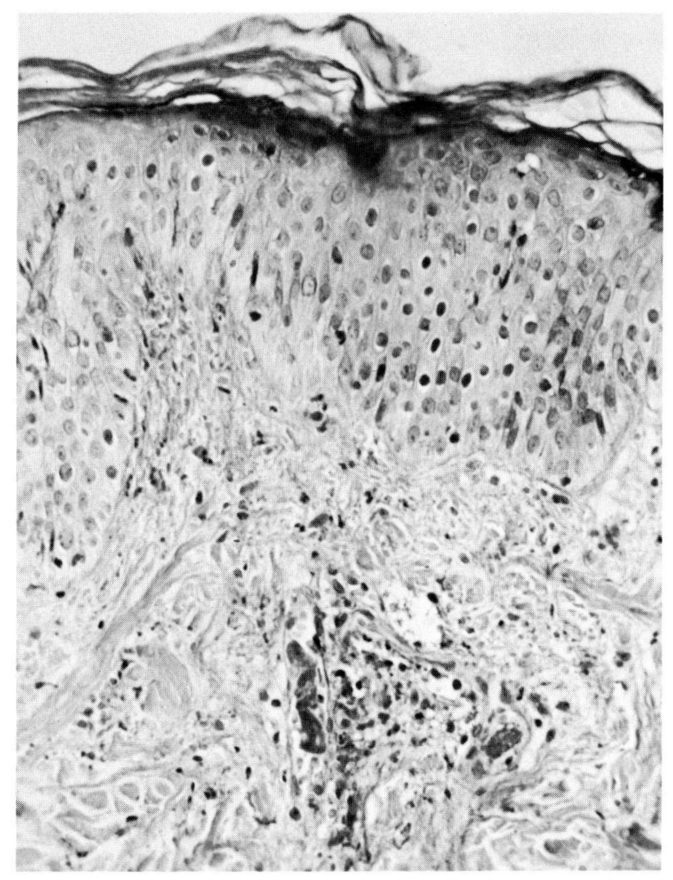

Figure X–14. Fibrin thrombus in a superficial vessel of the skin. There is extensive extravasation of red blood cells, but only scattered inflammatory cells. Case 3. (Hematoxylin and eosin stain, × 300.)

DIC may develop in addition to the primary disease. Thus findings of fibrin thrombi and inflammation may co-exist in these special cases. A more detailed discussion of differential features is presented elsewhere (173).

PATHOLOGY OF MAJOR BLOOD VESSELS

Large arteries and veins are involved in DIC in a large fraction (41%) of cases. This frequency was unexpected and previously such large vessel disease was a rarity in the

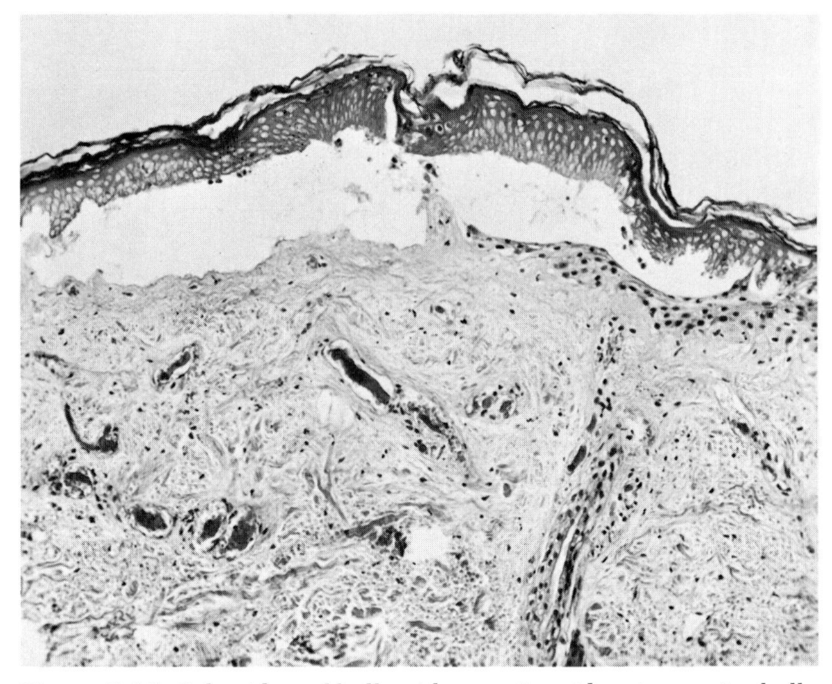

Figure X–15. Subepidermal bulla with necrotic epidermis covering bulla, nucleated squamous cells at margin of lesion (right), and fibrin thrombi plugging small venules. Case 6. (Hematoxylin and eosin stain, × 140.) (Robboy, Mihm, Colman, and Minna: *Br J Derm*, 88:221, 1973.)

literature. In part this is related to increasing use of vascular catheters for diagnostic and therapeutic maneuvers (49,140,214). Thrombotic occlusion frequently occurs about venous pressure catheters placed for measurement of central venous pressure or for cardiac pacing (Cases 8,33,38,43). The superior vena cava and basilic vein are most commonly affected. Three of our patients subsequently developed pulmonary emboli from these thrombotic sites (Cases 8,33,38). Arterial thrombi also develop at sites of manipulation, especially in arteries punctured for measurement of blood gases or those in which a catheter for blood pressure measurement are placed (Fig. X-22). Thrombosis can also occur as a complication of EACA therapy (119) (*see* Chap. XI-C) when fibrinolysis is inhibited. The following case illustrates the large vessel thrombosis that complicates catheter placement in veins and arteries in patients with DIC.

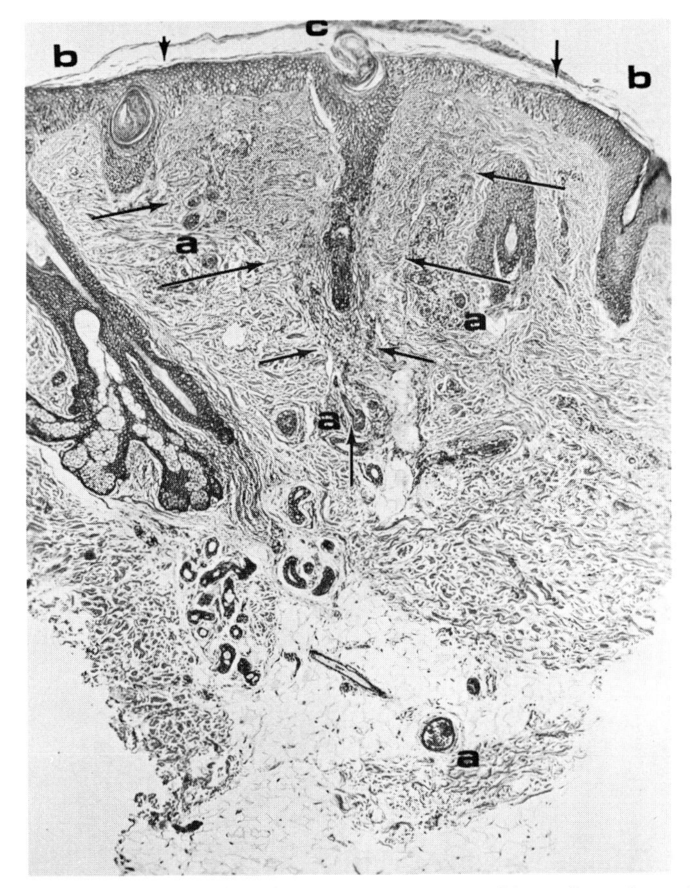

Figure X–16. Section petechiae of skin, showing fibrin thrombi in blood vessels (a), zone of hemorrhage (outlined by arrows), early epithelial necrosis, and incipient subepidermal bulla. Arrows demarcate the junction between normal (b) and involved (c) epidermis. Case 31. (Hematoxylin and eosin stain, × 50.) (Robboy, Colman, and Minna: *Hum Pathol, 3:*327, 1972.)

CASE 33 (TABLE X-III)—VIRAL MYOCARDITIS, SHOCK AND GANGRENE AT ARTERIAL CANNULATION SITE: A previously well 18-year-old male entered another hospital with dyspnea and a bilateral lower lobe pneumonia which was treated with penicillin. After six days he became cyanotic and went into shock and was treated with heparin for suspected deep vein thrombosis of the legs. He was transferred in a moribund state to the Massachusetts General Hospital.

He was febrile (101°F), in cardiogenic shock with hypotension (70 systolic, 50 diastolic), acidosis (pH 7.2), gallop rhythm, elevated venous pressure, pulmonary edema and oliguria (creatinine 2.8

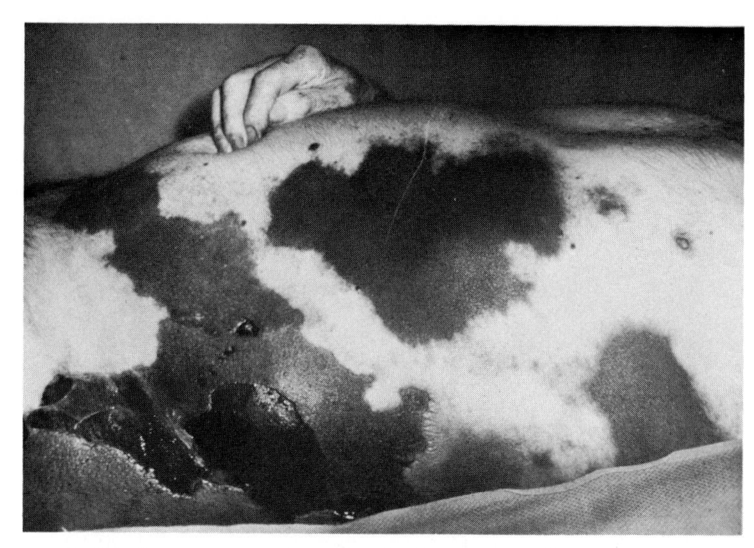

Figure X–17. Postmortem photograph, showing confluent purpura of varying ages (purpura fulminans). Case 6. (Colman and Kish: *N Engl J Med, 281:*153, 1969.)

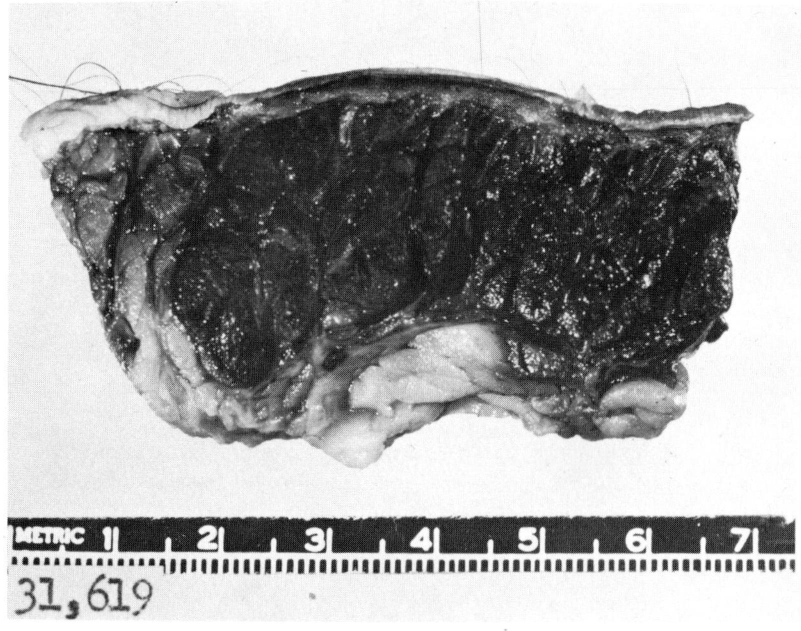

Figure X–18. Necrosis and hemorrhage of the full thickness of the skin from the patient in Figure X–17. (*Ibid.*)

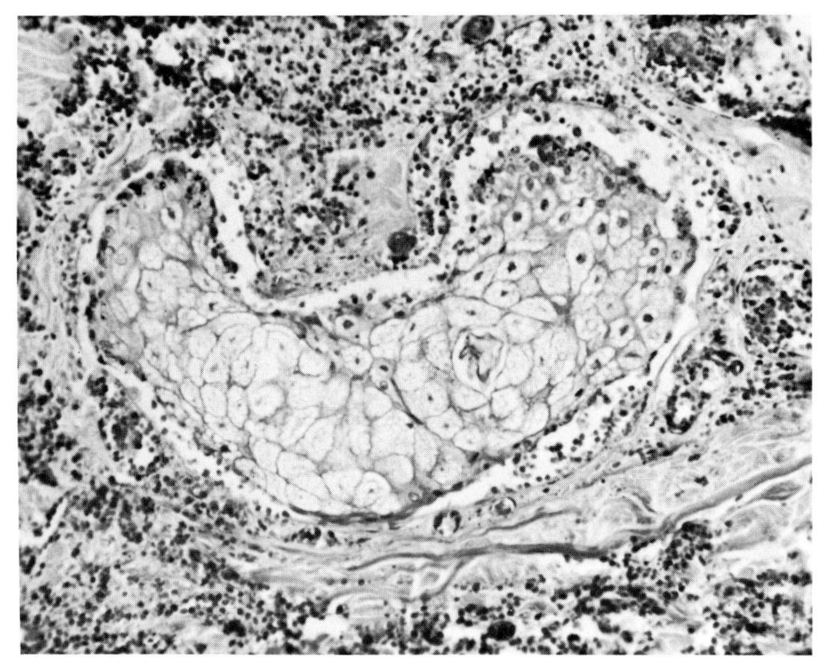

Figure X–19. Necrotic sebaceous gland and hemorrhage in skin. Case 6. (Hematoxylin and eosin stain, × 220.) (Robboy, Colman, and Minna: *Hum Pathol*, *3:*327, 1972.)

mg/dl). Mechanical ventilation was required for severe hypoxemia ($pO_2 50^{mmHg}$ on 100% FiO_2). See Table X-III for coagulation data. The SGOT was 950 units, LDH 790 units and CPK 54 units. Methylprednisolone, isoproterenal, morphine, diphenylhydantoin, and antibiotics were administered and heparin was stopped.

A catheter was placed in the left brachial artery to measure blood pressure. About twenty-four hours later, the left hand was blue and no pulses were felt. The arterial polyethylene catheter was removed. Because of persistent cyanosis of the fingers, the radial and ulnar arteries were exposed and clots removed. However, ten hours later, the left hand again became cold and cyanotic.

On the third hospital day upper gastrointestinal bleeding began and the hematocrit fell from 43% to 28%. At this time his basilic vein, in which the right atrial pacing catheter and central venous pressure catheter resided, became thrombosed. Suddenly, oozing of blood appeared at all venipuncture and cut-down sites. The coagulation tests were markedly abnormal. Heparin (3000 U every 4 hr) was administered. During the ensuing six hours the gastric, venipuncture and wound bleeding stopped and over the next day

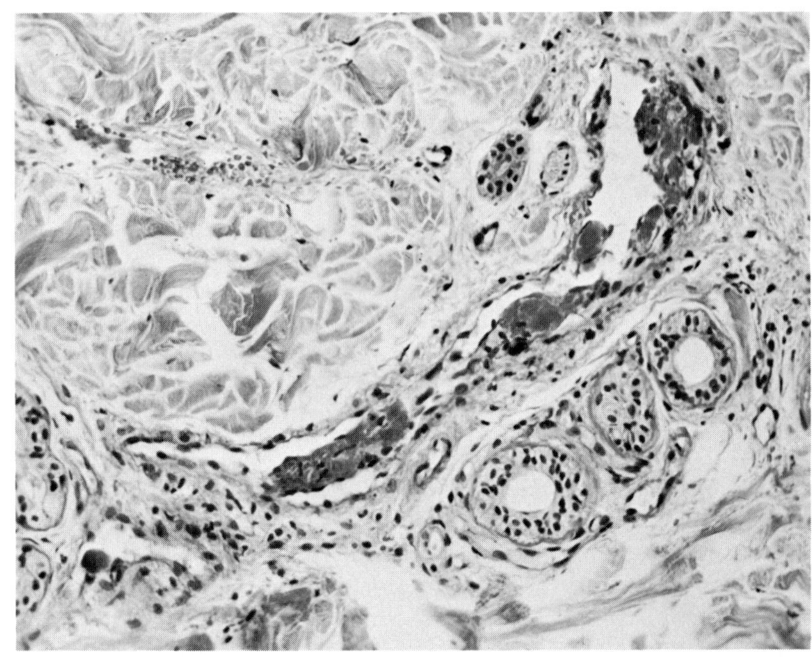

Figure X–20. Large thrombus of a major vessel of the deep reticular dermis of the skin. Case 6. (Hematoxylin and eosin stain, × 230.)

the coagulation tests improved. The tests for clotting function were all distinctly improved with the Fi dropping from 1:256 to 1:64 and the ELT rising from 3 to 15 min. EACA (8 gm loading dose, then 1 gm/hr IV) was then given. The CPK rose to 1470 units.

On the sixth hospital day the area of ischemic tissue in the left arm was sharply demarcated (Fig. X-23). On the next day, heparin and EACA were discontinued, the gangrenous left forearm was amputated and tracheostomy performed. Despite vigorous antibiotic and pressor therapy and correction of metabolic imbalance he went into coma two days later and developed progressive renal failure with cardiogenic shock. The tests of coagulation again became abnormal, and heparin (3000 U every 4 hr) was restarted. A diffuse petechial rash was present on the abdomen. Bleeding began from the tracheal suction, nasal, and oral mucous membranes. Death occurred. No virus could be identified in ante or postmortem material.

Autopsy revealed an extensive myocarditis and pneumonitis of probable viral origin. Fibrin thrombi were found in thirteen different organs including thrombosis of right brachial vein about catheter (Fig. X-24), a thrombus in superior vena cava about catheter tip (Fig. X-24) with acute pulmonary embolism probably as a secondary

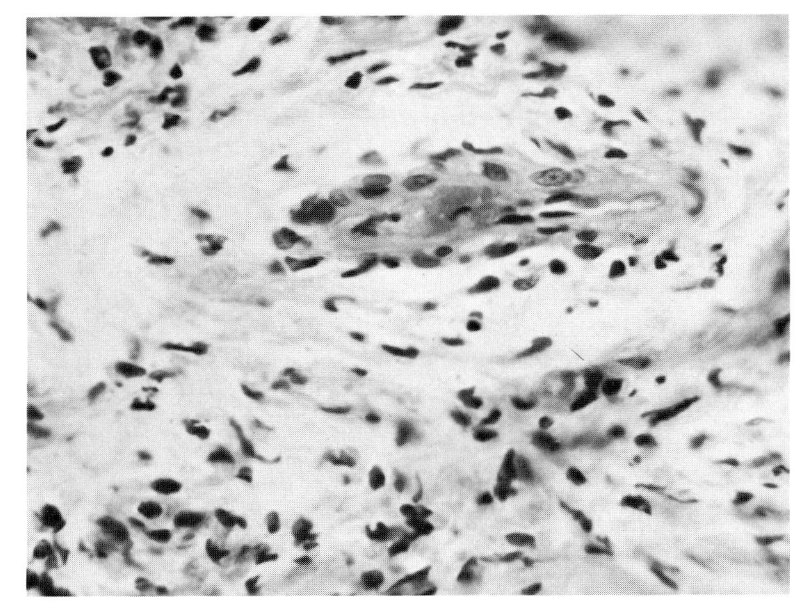

Figure X–21. Fibrin thrombus in a venule of the reticular dermis from a patient with gonococcemia. The chronic inflammatory reaction is a typical feature of the infectious disease process, but not of the DIC. Case 11. (Hematoxylin and eosin stain, × 630.)

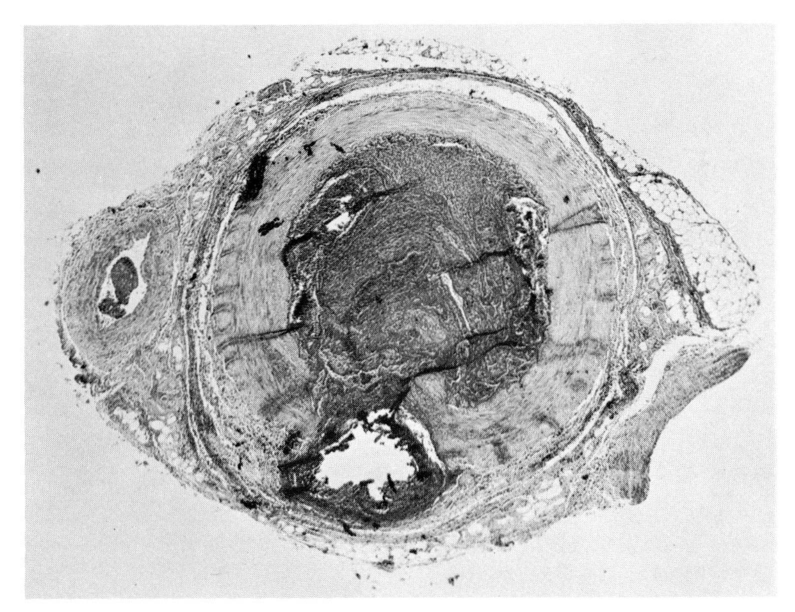

Figure X–22. Thrombosed radial artery in which a cannula had been temporarily placed. Case 43. (Hematoxylin and eosin stain, × 28.)

TABLE X-III
CASE 33

Time	Event	PT (sec)	Platelet count (per ul)	Fibrin-ogen (mg/dl)	PTT (sec)	ELT (min	Fi	Plasminogen (casein u/ml)
Admission	On heparin	nl	223,000	408	nl			
+ 3 day	Off heparin							
	Thrombosis	31	14,000	96		3	1 : 256	1.43
+ 4 day	On heparin	19	58,000	135	63	15	1 : 64	1.35
+ 6 day	Heparin +EACA	16	74,000	216	nl	nl	1 : 16	0.16
+ 7 day	Therapy stopped							
	Amputation arm	15	116,000	253	nl			
+ 9 day	DIC resume	17	20,000	168	53			

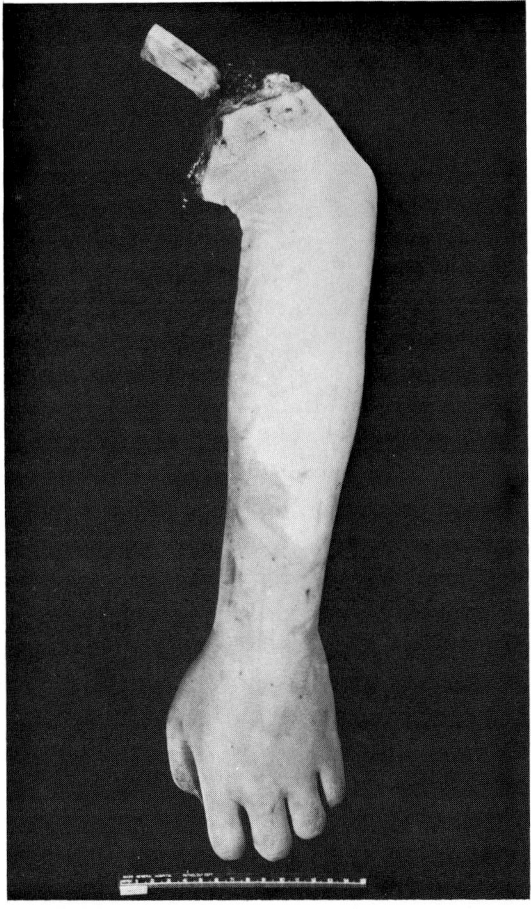

Figure X–23. Gangrene of arm caused by thrombosis of brachial artery about a catheter. Case 33. (*Ibid.*)

phenomenon, thrombophlebitis with thrombosis of popliteal veins (Fig. X-24), thrombosis of left radial artery secondary to catheter (surgical specimen) (Fig. X-23); and impending gangrene of toes.

Comment: This patient illustrates the danger of placing catheters in patients with DIC; the blood vessels may thrombose, causing gangrene and pulmonary embolism. This case also illustrates the association of DIC and systemic fibrinolysis. With one day of heparin therapy, both disease processes began to abate.

Thrombosis of major blood vessels also occurred as a complication of EACA therapy (*see* history of Case 15 in Chap. XI) or in systemic aspergillosis (*see* below).

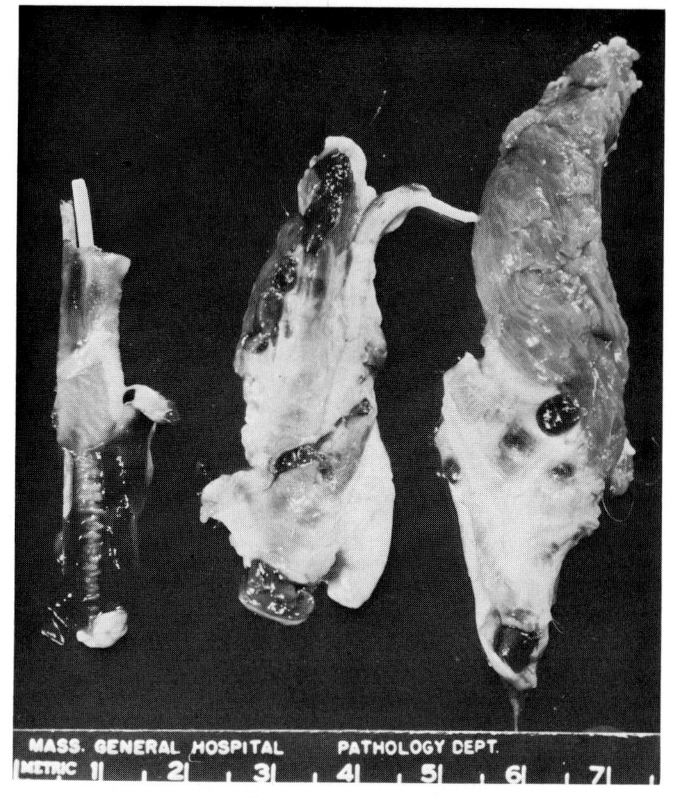

Figure X–24. Thrombosis of superior vena cava about a central venous pressure catheter and a cardiac pacing electrode (left), thrombosed basilic vein about a second catheter (middle), and popliteal veins with thrombophlebitis (right). Case 33.

ASPERGILLUS-INDUCED MICROANGIOPATHY AND DIC

As fungal infections become more prevalent in the increasing numbers of patients with impaired defense mechanisms, a syndrome of fungal invasion of blood vessels with resulting thrombosis, microangiopathy, leukoerythroblastosis and DIC is becoming apparent. The recognition of this syndrome is important as the fungal infection is often not recognized during life. The following two patients presented with leukoerythroblastosis, schistocytosis, coagulation test evidence for DIC and were found to have diffuse involvement of major arteries with aspergillus hyphae at necropsy (176, 181). *Candida albicans* appears to cause a similar syndrome (159).

CASE 28 (FIG. X-25)—SCHISTOCYTOSIS, HEMORRHAGIC DIATHESIS, RENAL FAILURE AND NEUROLOGIC SYMPTOMS MASQUERADING AS THROMBOTIC THROMBOCYTOPENIC PURPURA: A 66-year-old man entered the hospital with bruises and jaundice of eleven days' duration. Two weeks before admission chloramphenicol, tetracycline, erythromycin and prednisolone were prescribed for "influenza".

On admission, he was cachectic. Petechiae covered the arms, legs, and trunk, nontender ecchymoses, 2 to 4 cm in size, covered the forearms, right pectoral region, and legs and the stool was guaiac positive (4+).

The hematocrit was 23% and the WBC 9,600 with 70% neutrophils, 22% banded neutrophils, 5% metamyelocytes, and 3% myelocytes. In addition there were 32 normoblasts per 100 WBC. The peripheral blood smear disclosed an extraordinary number of schistocytes (Fig. VII-1). A bone marrow aspirate revealed marked erythroid hyperplasia and adequate number of normal

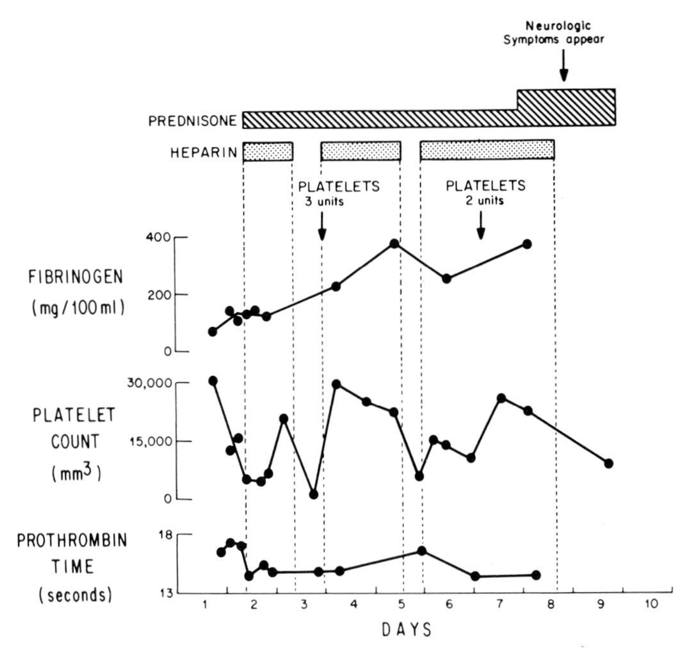

Figure X–25. Case 28. (Robboy, Salisbury, Ragsdale, Bobroff, Jacobson, and Colman: *Arch Intern Med, 128:*790, 1971).

megakaryocytes. The reticulocyte count was 9.4%, serum hemoglobin 23.2 mg/dl (normal, 2 to 3 mg/dl), and direct and indirect Coombs tests were negative. The tests of coagulation were abnormal (Fig. X-25). Cryofibrinogen was present.

Other laboratory studies included: BUN 126 mg, creatinine 3.1 mg, calcium 7.8 mg, phosphorus 6.3 mg, bilirubin 1.0 mg direct, and 2.6 mg/dl total, and lactic acid dehydrogenase 720 units. The urine sediment contained 10 RBC and 4 WBC/hpf and many coarsely granular pigmented casts. Multiple cultures of sputum, urine, blood and cerebrospinal fluid were negative. An X-ray film of the chest disclosed bilateral apical pleural scars and upward hilar retraction, but no infiltrates.

On admission several venipunctures were performed and within two hours, massive ecchymoses and bleeding developed at these sites, requiring transfusions. On the morning of the second day, gross hematuria developed and the stools became maroon. Therapy with heparin (6000 U every 4 hr) and prednisone (20 mg orally every 8 hr) was begun. By the next day the PT and the platelet count showed modest improvement and the heparin therapy was discontinued. When the platelet count suddenly fell, heparin therapy was reinstituted, 3 units of platelet concentrates were given, and during the next two days the platelet count and fibrinogen level improved. Again, the heparin was discontinued, and within six hours the platelet count and fibrinogen level fell, and the PT became prolonged. Heparin therapy was reinstituted at a constant infusion rate of 10 mg IV per hour.

During the sixth through the eighth days (while the patient was receiving heparin) results of the tests of hemostasis improved, and the bleeding slowed. The serum hemoglobin level fell to 10 mg/dl, and the number of schistocytes in the peripheral smears decreased markedly.

By the seventh day, the renal function was improved; the BUN was 50 mg and creatinine 1.5 mg/dl. Once rehydration was begun, the urine output averaged 2 to 3 liters per day. On the eighth day, in preparation for splenectomy, the dosage of prednisone was increased (to 40 mg orally every 6 hr) and the heparin therapy discontinued. At about this time, slight ptosis of the right eyelid and anisocoria were noted. By the morning of the tenth day the patient was obtunded, the gaze was disconjugated, flaccid paralysis developed in the left arm and leg, and death occurred.

Autopsy revealed *Aspergillus fumigatus* involving kidney (especially arcuate arteries), brain, heart, lung, thyroid, and spleen; fibrin thrombi in heart, pancreas, renal glomerular capillaries, and skin. Glomeruloid structures, a hallmark of TTP(205), were not observed.

Comment: This case, which was clinically indistinguishable from thrombotic thrombocytopenic purpura (TTP), is an example of aspergillus-induced microangiopathy and DIC.

CASE 45 (TABLE X-IV)—CIRRHOSIS, HEMORRHAGIC DIATHESIS AND MICROANGIOPATHY: A 15-year-old girl entered with a 9-month history consistent with postnecrotic cirrhosis. During the two weeks before admission bruises, epistaxes, black liquid stools, and ascites appeared. At admission she was disoriented, jaundiced, lethargic, had scattered ecchymoses on the hands and legs, petechiae dotting the body, and 4+ guaiac positive stool. The hematocrit was 35%, WBC 12,000, reticulocyte count 8.5%, and haptoglobin markedly decreased. The tests of clotting function were abnormal (Table X-IV). The conjugated bilirubin was 12 mg, the total bilirubin 22 mg/dl, total protein 5.5 gm (1.9 gm/dl albumin), SGOT 800 units, and alkaline phosphatase 5.2 units.

Therapy was begun with hydrocortisone, vitamin K and fresh whole blood and plasma. By the second day the ecchymoses enlarged; she was stuporous with bilateral decerebrate posturing, and the ammonia was > 150 ug/dl. The coagulation studies remained abnormal and the bilirubin rose to 30 mg/dl. On the eighth day she abruptly became alert, responded to commands and replied to questions.

Five days later a cut-down site on the left arm began oozing. The skin of the left antecubital fossa and palm was dark purple, necrotic and surrounded by hemorrhagic pustules. One day later, she was again stuporous, tachypneic and had perioral cyanosis. The fundus of the right eye became hemorrhagic.

The hematocrit was 30%, WBC 21,000 with 56% neutrophils, 37% band forms, 2% myelocytes and 1% late erythroblasts. Schistocytes were observed. The platelet count fell to 13,000/ul and the fibrinogen to 110 mg/dl. The conjugated bilirubin was 22 mg, total bilirubin 39 mg/dl and the SGOT 165. That evening bright red blood appeared from the rectum and in the oropharyngeal

TABLE X-IV
CASE 45

Day	PT (sec)	Platelet count	Fibrinogen (mg/dl)	TT (sec)	FDP
1	27	77,000	180		
2	23	112.000	140	33	1 : 16
3	24	89,000	170		
4	24			41	1 : 8
5	23				
6	24				
7	22				
8	24				
9	26		140		
10	24	45,000			
11	26	29,000		33	1 : 16
12	24	13,000			
13	26		110		
14	23	65,000	190	34	1 : 16

aspirate. Death occurred shortly thereafter. A culture of blood taken one day before death subsequently grew out aspergillus.

Autopsy showed postnecrotic cirrhosis, aspergillus septicemia involving skin, brain, heart, lung, esophagus, stomach, colon, and kidney (especially arcuate arteries). There were no varices in the esophagus.

Comment: This case is an example of aspergillus-induced microangiopathy and DIC.

In both cases the kidneys were enlarged. The cortices bulged with numerous hemorrhages, 1 to 3 cm in size (Fig. X-26), that corresponded to thrombosed arcuate arteries (Fig. X-27,28). Microscopically each thrombosed artery contained an intricate mesh of intertwined hyphae, some of which were anchored in the muscular wall. Filling the interstices of the hyphal trellis were thin fibrin strands (less than 1 μ in diameter) upon which red blood cells were caught, bent, and fragmented (Fig. X-29).

An *in vitro* model of Bull *et al.* (20) explains how red blood cells fragment as they are forcibly passed at high speeds through a fine mesh composed of thin fibers. The two essential facets are rapid blood flow, greater than 10 cm/sec, and obstructing fibers 1 μ or less in diameter. The composition of the fiber is immaterial; fibrin, glass, metal or nylon are equally effective. The present cases are presented as an *in vivo* example of this model. Aspergillus organisms, because of their abitlity to freely invade blood vessel walls, are able to anchor into arterial walls and form a network of interweaving hyphae in the lumina of the renal arteries (Fig. X-29). As fibrin-leukocyte-platelet thrombi form about the organisms, the two criteria for the model of Bull *et al.* (20) become fulfilled. *In vitro* aspergillus organisms alone neither cause hemolysis or elaborate a thromboplastic activity into serum (48).

ANALYSIS OF CAUSE OF DEATH

In our experience, DIC contributes strongly to patient mortality. Sixty-seven percent of patients (30/45) with DIC died in the hospital; in 60 percent of these patients the major cause of death was bleeding or thrombosis, especially in the

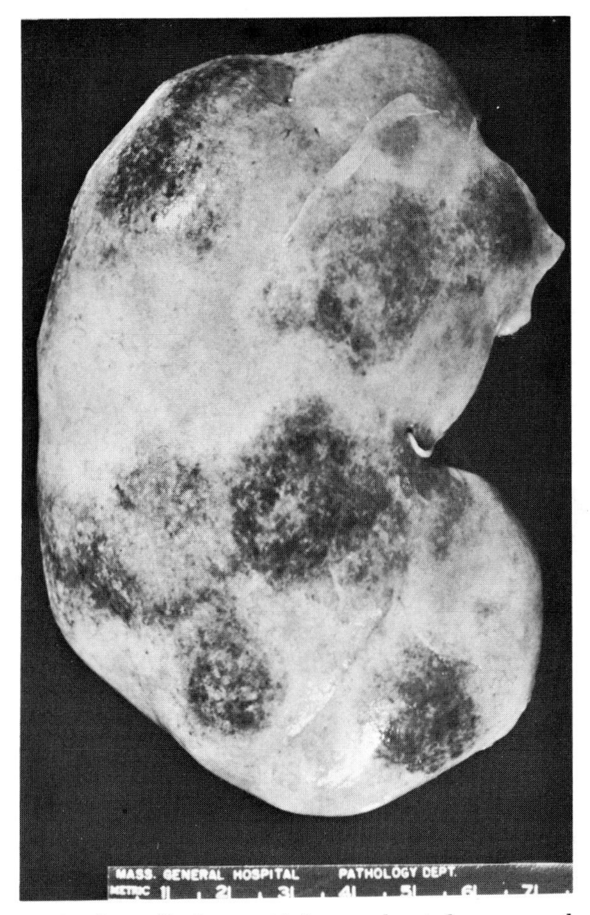

Figure X–26. Surface of kidney with hemorrhagic bosses, each representing an acute infarct. Case 28. (*Ibid.*)

lung, central nervous system, or gastrointestinal tract (Table X-V). In addition to major bleeding or thrombosis leading directly to death, three-quarters of the dying patients had some degree of bleeding and half had abnormal coagulation tests suggestive of ongoing DIC. However, we also stress the majority of the dying patients *had other factors* that were not directly attributable to DIC and that in themselves were major causes of death: pulmonary failure, prolonged hypotension, ongoing septicemia, renal and liver failure (Table X-V).

Pulmonary hemorrhage and edema apparently are directly

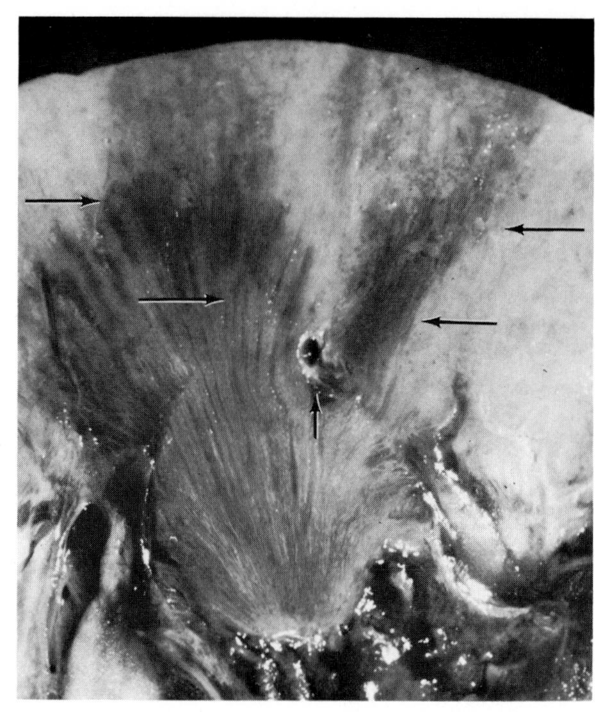

Figure X–27. Cut surface of kidney in Figure X–26 showing thrombosed arcuate artery and cortical infarct (arrows). Case 28. (*Ibid.*)

related to DIC as causes of death (*see* "Pulmonary dysfunction" in Chapter IX). Also, patients may have marked pulmonary hemorrhage associated with bronchopneumonia, neoplastic infiltrates or cardiac failure. These manifestations are probably causes of death related to DIC. The majority of hemorrhagic catastrophes involving the central nervous system are associated with infection or neoplastic infiltration. Thus when watching for signs of pulmonary or central nervous system hemorrhage, it is important to consider the primary disease processes that are present and their complications.

The assignment of DIC-induced thrombosis as a major cause of death is rarely straightforward. A patient may have diffuse eschars secondary to thrombosis of dermal vessels (purpura fulminans) and functionally lose his integument. This condition can be related directly to DIC and is analogous to a severe third degree burn. Thrombosis or embolic occlu-

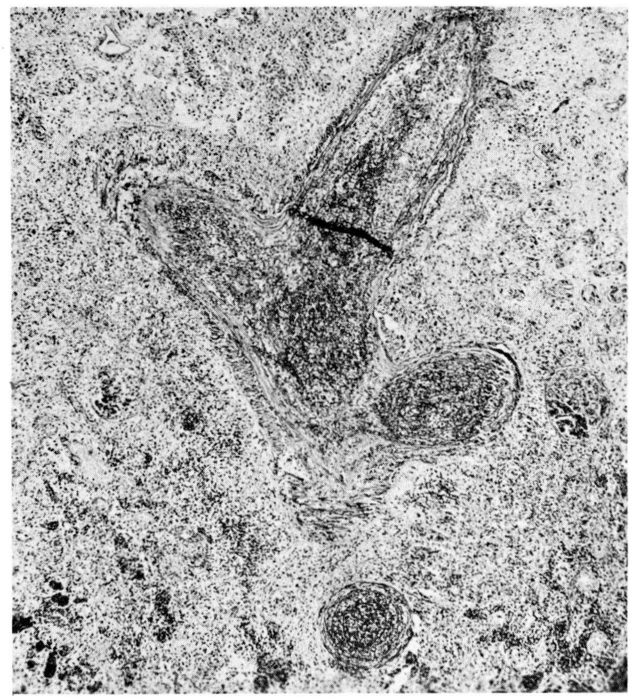

Figure X–28. Thrombosed arcuate artery of kidney. The aspergillus organisms are not seen with the hematoxylin and eosin stain. Case 28. (Hematoxylin and eosin stain, × 55.)

sion of central nervous system and pulmonary vessels occurs in patients with DIC, but in nearly all instances is associated with fungal infection, endocarditis, or intravascular catheters.

Prognostic Indicators in DIC

A few obvious factors appear to be significantly related to survival (Table X-VI). Patients who survived to leave the hospital generally have less severe bleeding, complete resolution of the underlying disease processes, and less abnormal coagulation tests at the time of diagnosis of DIC. Clinical manifestations associated with patients who died were: symptoms of pulmonary or central nervous system dysfunction, oliguria, greatly prolonged PT (> 25 sec) or severe hypofibrinogenemia (<100 mg/dl). Of interest, hypotension *per se* was not associated with decreased survival (Table V-II).

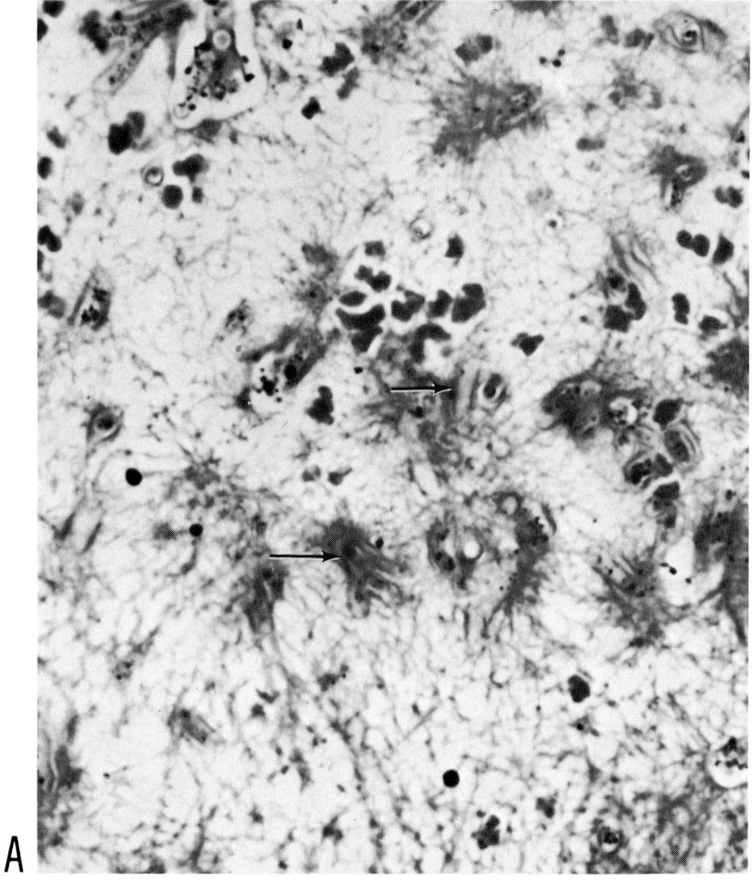

Figure X–29. Arcuate artery of kidney. Red blood cells are impinging upon fibrin strands that bridge the interstices among aspergillus hyphae (arrows). Case 28. (Swartz-Medrek-Robboy stain, × 820 (A), 1200 (B).) (Robboy, Colman, Minna: *Hum Pathol*, *3*:327, 1972.)

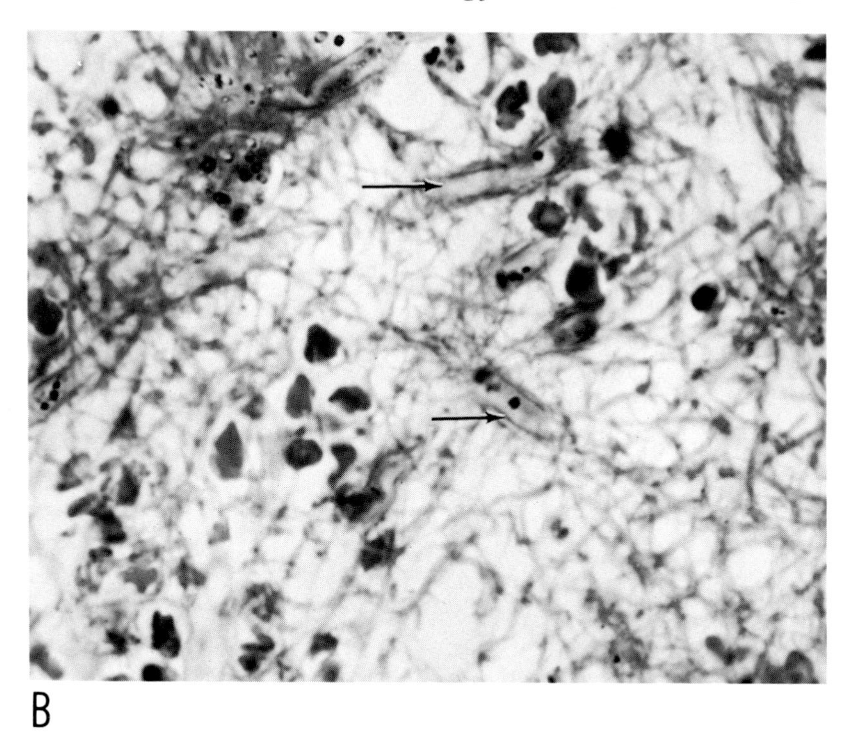

B

TABLE X-V

MAJOR CAUSES OF DEATH IN 30 PATIENTS WITH DIC[1]

CAUSES OF DEATH	# Patients	Frequency (%)	Case #
Major causes probably related to DIC (bleeding or thrombosis)	18	60	
Bleeding	14	47	
Bleeding into vital structures	10	33	
Lung, associated with:	8	28	
Pulmonary hemorrhage syndrome	5		12,16,21,27,29
Leukemic infiltrate[4]	1		5
Cardiac pulmonary edema	2		4,20
CNS, associated with:	5	18	
Aspergillus infection[4]	2		28,45
Leukemic infiltrate[4]	2		5,21
Unknown	1		4
Exsanguinating bleeding from GI tract	5	18	2,12,35,40,45
Thrombotic or embolic occlusion of major vessel	5	18	
Thrombosis in lung and CNS (Aspergillus)	2		28,45
Emboli[2]	3		1, 8,33
Diffuse skin thrombosis (75% of surface area)	1		6
Major causes not directly attributable to DIC[3]			
Pulmonary failure despite intubation	21	70	
Hypotension, > 1 day	16	53	
Ongoing septicemia	16	53	
Cardiogenic shock	10	33	
Severe acute renal failure	7	23	12,15,19,25,32,33,34
Liver failure	4	13	4,37,40,45

[1] Postmortem examination performed in 22/30 patients.

[2] Emboli: Case #8, CNS from marantic endocarditis; Case #33, lung from catheters in superior vena cava; Case #1, lung from inferior vena cava thrombosis.

[3] Cases with pulmonary and exsanguinating hemorrhage were excluded from categories of pulmonary failure and hypotension.

[4] Destruction of blood vessels by the primary disease may be the more important cause of bleeding.

TABLE X-VI
PROGNOSTIC INDICATORS IN DIC

LABORATORY		During DIC			After Therapy			CLINICAL		
	N	PT	Platelets	Fibrinogen	PT	Platelets	Fibrinogen	Overall Severity of Bleeding	#of Bleeding Sites	Survival (leave hospital)
Died of bleeding or thrombosis	14	−								
Died during episode of DIC	21	−		−−	−	−	−−	+	+	
Survived	17	+	+	++	+	++	−−	−−−		
Complete resolution of underlying disease	13	+	+	+++					−−−	+++
Bleeding stopped	21	+	+++	++	+++	++	++			++

Symbols indicate the occurrence of significant differences between the indicated patient groups and the remainder of the patients: Blank, no significant difference; + or −, $P < 0.05$; ++ or −−, $P < 0.01$; +++ or −−−, $P < 0.001$. The + symbols indicate a higher or more normal laboratory value, while − symbols indicate the opposite. In the case of clinical observations + symbols indicate: more severe bleeding, greater number of bleeding sites, more units transfused, a longer duration or higher incidence of survival while − symbols indicate the opposite.

In summary, bleeding and thrombosis play a major role in the mortality of DIC; however, most patients had other processes sufficient in themselves to cause death. Signs of pulmonary or central nervous system hemorrhage or thrombosis in patients with DIC have an ominous prognosis. The degree of bleeding and coagulation test abnormalities can predict survival in patients with DIC. Patients with severe bleeding, very prolonged PT and severe hypofibrinogenemia also have an ominous prognosis.

PROBLEM-ORIENTED APPROACH TO AUTOPSY

An autopsy that has been carefully performed and the findings correlated with the clinical history may yield much information about the pathogenesis and natural history of DIC. Table X-VII presents a problem-oriented approach by which the autopsy might be performed when DIC is suspected. The corresponding problem-oriented approaches that deal with the history, physical examination, and laboratory studies are presented in Chapter XIV.

The autopsy should begin with careful gross inspection of the skin, other external tissues such as eyes and mouth, and then the internal organs and body cavities. If petechiae, purpura, palpable variants of both, or gangrene are found in the skin, microscopical sections should be prepared. Catheters, if present during the external examination, should be left *in situ* so that the appropriate major blood vessels can be examined for thrombosis.

Hemorrhage into lungs is often due to underlying disease processes such as bronchopneumonia or leukemic infiltrates, but not infrequently it may be out of proportion to the underlying disease and may be secondary to DIC. The brain, kidneys, and heart should be examined for intrinsic diseases that may give rise to signs of organ dysfunction. Since liver disease, especially cirrhosis, gives rise to abnormal coagulation values, it is important at autopsy to ascertain the status of this organ.

Organs frequently contain fibrin thrombi, but appear grossly to be normal at autopsy. Thus, multiple sections of the kidney and at least one section of the adrenal, choroid plexus of the brain, liver, lung, and testis should be prepared

TABLE X-VII

PROBLEM ORIENTED APPROACH TO A PATIENT WITH SUSPECTED DIC: BIOPSY AND AUTOPSY

Signs of bleeding:
- Skin: petechiae, purpura, palpable purpura, hemorrhagic bullae, acral gangrene, purpura fulminans
- External and internal examination: conjunctiva, mucosal linings
- Into body cavities: pleural, peritoneal, pericardial, gastrointestinal, central nervous system

Organs that specifically should be examined grossly:
- Major blood vessels: is there thrombosis about catheters?
- Kidney: renal cortical necrosis (Shwartzman phenomenon)
- Liver: is there intrinsic damage (cirrhosis, hepatitis)?
- Lung: is hemorrhage out of proportion to underlying disease? Pulmonary emboli, source

Organs that should be routinely examined microscopically for fibrin thrombi:
- Kidney, multiple sections
- Adrenal
- Brain, choroid plexus
- Liver
- Lung
- Testis
- Bone marrow examination

Organ dysfunction:
- Evidence of intrinsic disease to account for clinical signs or symptoms: atherosclerosis, bronchopneumonia, nephrosclerosis, cirrhosis?

Cause of death:
- Identify all underlying disease operative at time of death
- Evidence of ongoing hemostatic abnormalities at time of death
  - Coagulation tests abnormal?
  - Exsanguination, into body cavity?
- Evidence of thrombosis of major vessels.
- Factors not caused or rarely caused by DIC: pulmonary failure, hypotension, septicemia, cardiogenic shock, acute renal failure (tubular necrosis), hepatic failure.

for microscopic examination. Examination of the bone marrow may provide information regarding the potential platelet and red cell production.

Lastly, the autopsy helps to ascertain why a patient has died, whether death was related to DIC or some other process, the effect of therapy, and whether iatrogenic or therapeutic maneuvers can be implicated. Not infrequently, unexpected exsanguination into a body cavity causes death. More frequently, however, death is due to pulmonary failure, hypertension, septicemia, cardiogenic shock, acute tubular necrosis, or hepatic failure, despite ongoing hemostatic abnormalities. The autopsy suggests commonly that DIC is already under control at the time of death, but that death was related to an unremitting underlying disease process.

CHAPTER XI

RESPONSE TO THERAPY

THERAPY OF A PATIENT WITH DIC is complex, since the diseases which underlie the DIC, the additional precipitating factors present, and the biochemical systems that have been triggered must all be considered. Possible therapy includes correction of underlying diseases (e.g. septicemia), other precipitating factors (e.g. acidosis), hemostatic defects not due to DIC (e.g. vitamin K deficiency), replacement of blood components, and use of drugs which inhibit the coagulation (e.g. heparin) or fibrinolytic (e.g. EACA) systems. This chapter presents criteria for clinical and laboratory evaluation of the efficacy of therapy and the effects of various regimens.

CRITERIA FOR RESPONSE TO THERAPY

The obvious overall goal of therapy is for the patient to return to a normal state of health, or at a minimum to the state prior to the DIC. However, patients with DIC often have many coexisting pathologic processes, which makes it difficult to objectively evaluate the clinical response of DIC to treatment in such a complex situation. We have found that a set of criteria which can be applied at the bedside and which relies on tests routinely available in the average clinical laboratory is of great value in assessing the severity of DIC and whether or not it has been brought under control.

The criteria for response of the hemorrhagic-thrombotic manifestations and coagulation tests are listed in Table XI-I. A patient was considered improved if bleeding ceased or thromboses became no problem in management or threat to survival, and the coagulation tests improved.

The categories of unchanged or worse are clinically obvious. Because the platelet count responds more slowly than the other coagulation tests, improvement in throm-

TABLE XI-I

CRITERIA FOR RESPONSE OF DIC TO THERAPY

Combined clinical and coagulation criteria	
Improved	Bleeding completely stops, acral cyanosis disappears All coagulation tests (except platelet count) improve
Partial	Major bleeding stops, acral cyanosis disappears At least two coagulation tests improve
Unchanged	Bleeding or acral cyanosis unchanged
Worse	Bleeding, purpura, acral cyanosis increase or new thromboses appear Coagulation tests worse (if bleeding unchanged)
Indeterminate	Death in < 24 hours
Coagulation tests[1]	
Prothrombin time	Return to normal, or > 5 sec fall
Fibrinogen	Rise of > 40 mg/dl
Platelets	Rise by > 50,000/ul; if absolute count < 50,000/ul, rise by 100%
FDP (Fi)	Fall by titer of ≥ 4 (≥ 2 tube dilutions)
Euglobulin lysis	Return to normal

[1] Coagulation values are given only for improvement; to be scored as worse, the same quantitative changes apply but in opposite direction.

bocytopenia was not made a requirement for complete improvement. Patients living less than 24 hours after initiation of therapy for an episode of DIC are classified as indeterminant for bleeding response.

All relevant forms of therapy directed against DIC, fibrinolysis or the underlying primary disease are summarized for each patient in Table I-III. Regardless of the form of therapy, a significant length of time (average 3 to 4 days) usually elapses before the bleeding slows or stops (Table XI-II). In the majority of instances the PT and fibrinogen values do not maximally improve until a similar period has elapsed. The platelet count gives variable results and in over half the patients with complete cessation of bleeding requires more than a week to respond.

The coagulation tests at the time of diagnosis of DIC have predictive value regarding the bleeding response, while clinical assessment of hemorrhagic severity has less. At the time of diagnosis of DIC, the PT, platelets and fibrinogen are significantly less abnormal in those patients whose bleeding eventually stops compared with those whose bleeding will be unchanged or worse. However, these groups are not distinguishable by: number of bleeding sites, fall in hematocrit, transfusion requirement, or presence of hypotension.

Similarly, there is significant correlation between improvement in coagulation tests and cessation of bleeding. Normal prothrombin time values and high fibrinogen levels were achieved by these patients who stopped bleeding; while the platelet count on the average rose, it was still significantly lower than normal (Table XI-II).

HEPARIN THERAPY

Pharmacology

Since most of the characteristic clinical and laboratory findings of DIC can be conceptually regarded as results of thrombin activity, it would seem logical that the therapy of DIC should be focused in part on blocking the actions of this proteolytic enzyme. The most potent, reliable, and effective antagonist of thrombin is heparin, a substance that occurs naturally in the liver and lung, but for which no physiological role is known. Heparin is not demonstrable in the systemic circulation, and no pathological condition has yet been reported in which excess heparin has been implicated.

Heparin is a unique mucopolysaccharide with a high content of sulfate groups (2.5 per disaccharide unit). It is the strongest organic acid which naturally occurs and can be injected into man safely. It possesses the highest negative electric charge of any biologically active compound, and can

TABLE XI-II
COAGULATION TESTS AND BLEEDING STATUS
AFTER ALL TYPES OF THERAPY[1]

Bleeding Status	No. of Episodes	PT (Sec)	Platelets	Fibrinogen (mg/dl)	Time[2] days
Completely stops	20	13.5	100,000	314	3.1
Major bleeding stops	7	18.5	73,000	275	3.4
Unchanged or worse	13	19.5	39,000	167	5.2

[1] If computed for therapy with heparin alone, the values are similar.
[2] Average time for bleeding response to occur, or time of observation in patients with unchanged or worse bleeding.

therefore interfere with a wide variety of biochemically important reactions in which proteins are involved.

Although heparin inhibits more than twenty different enzyme systems *in vitro,* it has only two known functions *in vivo:* activation of lipoprotein lipase, and anticoagulant activity. Heparin profoundly inhibits various stages of the coagulation system. In concert with a plasma co-factor, antithrombin III, its cardinal action is the inhibition of thrombin. All actions of thrombin are thereby inhibited, including fibrin monomer formation and the thrombin-related-activation of factors VIII, V and XIII. Heparin also directly blocks the proteolytic activity of factor Xa (219,220). Thus heparin is theoretically an ideal drug to block the action of thrombin and by inference the syndrome of DIC.

Heparin Dosage

Once the decision is made to treat a patient with heparin, it should be given intravenously every four hours in doses ranging from 3000 to 10,000 USP units. Doses for children must be calculated on a per kilogram basis. With increasing doses of heparin, the fibrinogen rises (average 4.3 fold), while the platelet count and PT change only slightly (Fig. XI-1).

Monitor of Heparin-anticoagulant Activity

The whole blood clotting time can be used to monitor the anticoagulation effect of heparin. Although the PTT is a more accurate test of heparin anticoagulation than the clotting time when the hemostatic system is intact (35), it is unreliable in DIC. A prolonged PTT during therapy cannot discriminate between changes in the effects of heparin and the factor depletion and anticoagulant effect of FDP associated with DIC. Thus, a PTT which suddenly becomes more prolonged during therapy cannot distinguish overheparinized patients from the patient with acutely worse DIC.

The insensitivity of the whole blood clotting time to low factor levels and moderately high FDP titers make this test the most suitable control for heparin. From experience with

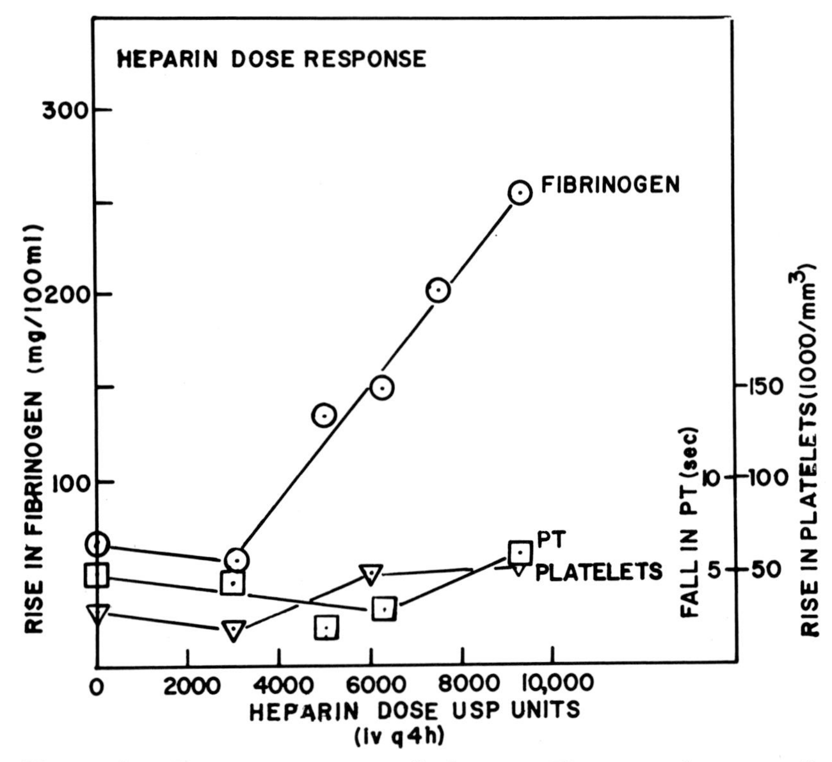

Figure XI–1. Dose response curve for heparin. The mean changes in fibrinogen, platelet count, and PT were calculated for four to ten patients per point, and plotted as a function of heparin dose.

anticoagulant therapy in deep vein thrombosis a reasonable therapeutic endpoint is prolongation of the clotting time to two to three times the normal control. Because DIC may be severe or because patients may initially show heparin resistance, large doses of heparin frequently have to be administered for several days to achieve therapeutic clotting times.

Similarly, some patients who have ongoing DIC and are improving while receiving heparin, may suddenly develop a reexacerbation of their DIC, manifest by the expected clinical and laboratory criteria, and also in part by a fall in the clotting time. Increasing the heparin dosage results again in therapeutic clotting times and control of the DIC (*see* history of Case 13, Chap. VI). As patients improve, the heparin requirement decreases. The heparin dosage can be adjusted to the clotting time, so as to prevent overheparinization.

Results of Heparin Therapy

Over half of our patients (54%) showed improvement in their clinical and coagulation test status after heparin therapy was begun (Tables XI-III and IV). This usually required an average of three days of therapy. Over two thirds of these patients also survived to leave the hospital.

Of special interest are patients who some might classify as having fibrinolysis on the basis of the initial coagulation data. Patients (Cases 13,24,33,37) with abnormal ELTs, low plasminogen levels, elevated titers of FDP, or whole clot lysis (Cases 14,16A) have been treated with heparin alone. All showed clinical and coagulation test improvement (Table I-III). In five of these six patients the basic underlying diseases remained unchanged. Thus, heparin therapy alone was associated with cessation of the manifestations of fibrinolysis (*see also* "Systemic Fibrinolysis," Chap. VI).

Possible Complications of Heparin Therapy

Serious complications of heparin therapy in DIC are uncommon (one of twenty-six patients in this series) (*see* Case 17 below). However, a large percentage (60%) of patients develop increased bleeding within the first two days of heparin therapy, but most stop bleeding even though the heparin is continued (average time 2.9 days after starting heparin). During the period of increased bleeding the patients have deteriorating coagulation tests (rising PT, falling platelets, falling fibrinogen), indicating that ongoing DIC rather than heparin overdosage has caused the bleeding. Although all new episodes of bleeding should be reevaluated in patients with DIC, this phenomenon of continued or increased bleeding during the early phase of therapy should be recognized.

CASE 17—MENINGITIS, HEPARIN THERAPY, AND SUBDURAL HEMORRHAGE OF THE SPINAL COLUMN: A 9-year-old girl entered with meningismus and fever (107° F). During the previous week she had received penicillin for a sore throat. On admission the blood pressure was 80 systolic, 60 diastolic and nonpalpable petechiae were present on the ankles, soft palate, forearm and trunk. The peripheral blood contained numerous helmet and burr shaped red cells. The PT was 15 sec, platelets 9000/ul, and fibrinogen 100

TABLE XI-III
RESPONSE TO THERAPY OF BLEEDING PATIENTS BY COMBINED CLINICAL AND COAGULATION CRITERIA

Therapy	# of patients[1]	# of Episodes[2]	Improved	Improved partial	Unchanged	Worse	Indeterminate	Survive
Heparin	24	28	14	5	2	1	6	9
Heparin + EACA	4	5	1	3	0	1	0	1
EACA	3	4	0	1	0	3	0	2
None	10	13	3	1	0	6	3	3

[1] Initial episode only tabulated for patients with multiple episodes.

[2] See Table XI-I for combined criteria, and Tables I-II, III for individual patient data. Four episodes (9, 11, 22, 39) with no bleeding or thrombotic manifestations are not included in this table, but their associated coagulation data are included in Table XI-IV.

TABLE XI-IV

DETAILED ANALYSIS OF RESPONSE TO THERAPY[1]

(Number of Episodes)

THERAPY	No. of Patients[2]	*CLINICAL BLEEDING-ACROCYANOSIS*					*LABORATORY*														
							PT			*PLATELETS*			*FIBRINOGEN*			*FI*			*ELT*		
		Imp	PI	NC	W	Ind	Imp	NC	W	Imp	NC	W	Imp	NC	W	Imp	NC	W	Imp	NC	W
Heparin	26	15	4	3	1	6	15	4	2	7	13	1	21	1	0	10	1	1	6	1	0
Heparin + EACA	5	1	3	0	1	0	1	3	1	1	3	1	5	0	0	0	1	0	1	0	1
EACA	4	1	0	2	1	0	0	0	3	0	1	3	1	1	1	0	0	0	1	0	0
None	15	3	1	3	6	3	3	5	0	3	5	1	5	2	0	1	1	0	1	0	0

[1] Imp, improved; PI, partially improved; NC, no change; W, worse; Ind, indeterminate. See Table XI-I for criteria.

[2] The number of individual patients in each treatment group. The number of total episodes in each treatment group were: heparin, 29; heparin + EACA, 5; EACA, 4; none, 16. The patients without bleeding or acrocyanosis are scored under the no change category of clinical response.

mg/dl. The hematocrit was 33%, WBC 9600/ul, and the spinal fluid contained numerous neutrophils and lymphocytes; no organisms were seen and all cultures were sterile. Penicillin and sulfisoxazole were administered.

Twelve hours after admission, hematemesis occurred and the PT was 24 sec, platelets 3000/ul, Fi titer 1:160, and ELT normal. Whole blood and heparin (3125 units every 4 hr) were given. After four units of platelets, serial counts revealed a half-disappearance time of 6–10 hours. During the next two days she received an additional 8 units of platelets and the clotting time increased from 31 to 51 min, the Fi titer rose further to 1:1280, and the fibrinogen to 320 mg/dl. At this time a febrile transfusion reaction occurred and the serum haptoglobin was decreased.

On the fifth hospital day hydrocortisone (100 mg IV every 9 hr) was started. Nuchal rigidity and mid-back pain developed, followed by anisocoria, papilledema, multiple retinal hemorrhages of the right eye, paraplegia, anesthesia from T-10 downward, and urinary retention. The platelets were 38,000/ul and fibrinogen 340 mg/dl. The heparin was stopped, protamine sulfate (25 mg IV) administered, and hydrocortisone increased (100 mg IV every 6 hr). Seven units of platelets were given and serial platelet counts revealed a half-disappearance time of 3–7 hours. Five hours later the papilledema cleared and the pupils became equal. At laminectomy, a subdural hematoma was found to extend from T-10 to L-4.

During the next two weeks the platelets rose to 390,000/ul and the fibrinogen to 400 mg/dl. No further bleeding occurred but she remained paraplegic and was discharged on the sixtieth day.

Comment: The major question concerns whether the subdural hematoma formed because of heparin, the DIC, or the unchecked meningitis. The fibrinogen level had risen from 100 to 340 mg/dl at the time of hematoma formation and the coagulation tests did not deteriorate when protamine was administered. However, the Fi titer had shown a progressive rise and serial platelet counts demonstrated a rapid consumption of platelets immediately preceding the development of the hematoma. It is possible that the transfusion reaction and platelet administration aggravated the DIC. The prolongation of clotting time could have been secondary to either heparin overdose, or to ongoing DIC. It was impossible to definitively establish the etiology of the hematoma.

EPSILON-AMINO CAPROIC ACID (EACA) THERAPY ALONE

EACA is a drug that resembles lysine except for the absence of the alpha-amino group. It is a non-specific inhibitor of plasmin, and EACA at high concentrations almost totally inhibits the activation of plasminogen (3). The drug is completely absorbed orally. The recommended oral dose is 4 gm every 4 hours. When the drug is administered intravenously, the loading dose is 4 gm followed by a continuous infusion of 1 gm every hour (121).

EACA has been employed extensively when fibrinolysis has been considered the cause of or a factor contributing to hemorrhage (151). At the present time, however, the indications for its systemic use are limited. EACA has also been used in the treatment of hemophilia (122), but a well-controlled study has failed to indicate it has any value (195).

The major indication for the use of EACA is in the control of bleeding in the urinary tract. Since it is filtered but not reabsorbed by the kidney, high levels result in the urine. It inhibits urokinase and thus blocks localized urinary tract fibrinolysis. Thus, EACA is effective in controlling the hematuria that occurs after prostatic surgery (120). EACA also appears to effectively terminate hematuria in hemophiliacs (191), but large clots may develop, leading to urinary obstruction.

Other experimental actions of the drug include delay of homograft rejection (69) and inhibition of delayed hypersensitivity (110). Since EACA also inhibits the complement system (197), it has been used with some effectiveness in hereditary angioneurotic edema (63).

EACA therapy may also have adverse effects. Massive necrosis and myoglobinuria (95) may occur after long term therapy, but the complication is rare.

Probably, the single entity in which EACA therapy can be predictably expected to result in complications, sometimes fatal, is the fibrinolysis secondary to DIC. When EACA is given to patients with DIC without concurrent heparin administration, thrombotic complications sometimes ensue (76,79,141,168).

Since the action of EACA is to inhibit fibrinolysis, the EACA would be expected to be useful in conditions where the fibrinolysis was primary, or where the DIC was local and bleeding at the local site was due to the activated fibrinolytic system (e.g. Case 23). In actuality there are very few patients who fall into the category of having "primary fibrinolysis", an observation made by McKay (116), Merskey *et al.* (130) and confirmed by our experience.

The following two cases (#15,10) are examples of complications of EACA therapy.

CASE 15 (FIGS. XI-2–4)—AORTIC SURGERY, FIBRINOLYSIS, AND THROMBOSIS FOLLOWING EACA THERAPY: A 61-year-old hypertensive white female entered with interscapular pain. The PT was 13 sec and platelets 754,000/ul. On the third day, a large fusiform dissecting aneurysm which extended from vertebrae T5-T10 was resected and replaced with a teflon graft. At the time the aortic clamps were removed, the heart-lung pump was stopped, and protamine sulfate was given (to neutralize the effect of heparin). Only three units of blood had been required during the procedure.

Thirty minutes later massive bleeding appeared throughout the thoracic cavity. She was transfused with 20 units of whole blood (4 fresh) during a one hour period. The PT was 16 sec, PTT 36 sec, platelets 184,000/ul, fibrinogen 350 mg/dl, TT 23 sec, ELT 5 min and Fi 1:16.

EACA (5 g IV loading dose, then 1 gm IV every hour) was administered and the bleeding dramatically stopped. One hour later the PT was 17 sec and platelets 98,000/ul. Twenty hours postoperatively she developed a phrenic nerve palsy, flaccid paraplegia of both legs, and anesthesia to a level of vertebra T4. The PT, PTT, thrombin time, and ELT were normal. The platelets were 69,000/ul and fibrinogen 310 mg/dl. The EACA was stopped and heparin (6000 U every 4 hr) was started.

However, the paraplegia remained constant throughout the remainder of the hospital course. She developed progressive respiratory failure and died on the seventh postoperative day.

Autopsy showed that the spinal cord was infarcted from T10 distally (Fig. XI-2). Several vessels, including the anterior median spinal artery (Fig. XI-3), the central arteries and occasionally a vessel of the anterior pial plexus contained fibrin thrombi (Fig. XI-4). Other findings included acute bronchopneumonia, atherosclerosis, and cardiomegaly.

Comment: This case is presented as a complication of EACA therapy in which "primary fibrinolysis" was inhibited with EACA, unmasking DIC, and leading to fatal thrombosis.

CASE 10 (FIG. XI-5)—CIRRHOSIS, GRAM NEGATIVE SEPTICEMIA AND COAGULATION CHANGES AFTER SEQUENTIAL HEPARIN, EACA, AND HEPARIN THERAPY AGAIN: A 32 year old man with a history of alcoholism entered with diffuse purpura of three days' duration. Two months previously the PT was 19 sec and the platelets 56,000/ul. One week before admission, chills, nausea and vomiting

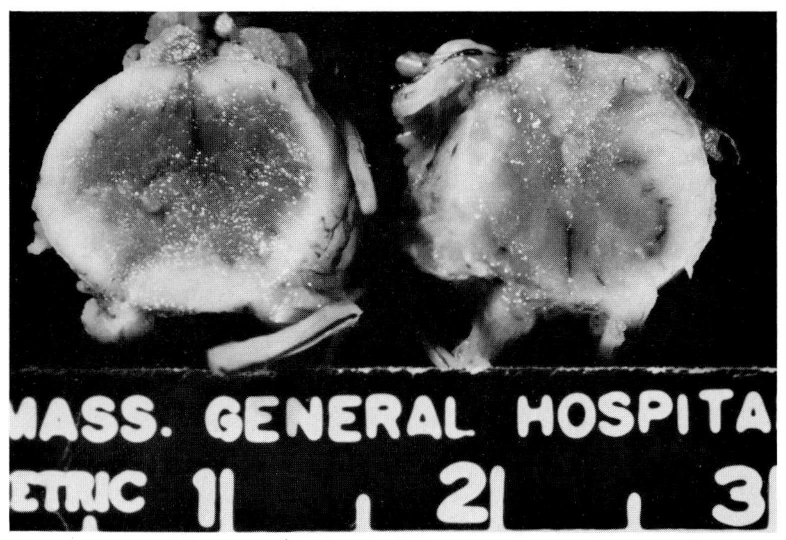

Figure XI–2. Spinal cord infarct. Case 15. (Robboy, Colman, Minna: *Hum Pathol, 3*:327, 1972.)

occurred followed by the purpuric eruption. Physical examination revealed stigmata of Laennec's cirrhosis. In addition, the various types of skin lesions including bleeding, bullous and crusted erosions of the lips and nasal mucosa and palpable 0.5 cm. purpura on the palms, chest, and legs. A gram stain of a skin lesion showed multiple gram negative intracellular diplococci. Multiple cultures were negative. Therapy was begun with penicillin, methicillin, vitamins, and folic acid.

On the second day the platelets fell, and the PT rose (Fig. XI-5). Gross hematuria appeared and heparin (6200 U every 4 hr) was started. One day later all tests of clotting function returned partially towards normal. EACA (5 gm loading dose, then 1 gm IV hourly) was added.

On the seventh day, the tests of clotting function were only mildly abnormal but the bilirubin was 23 mg/dl. The heparin and antibiotics were discontinued but the EACA continued. During the ensuing three days, the PT rose from 19 to 27 sec, whereas the platelets fell from 197,000 to 63,000/ul and the fibrinogen from 194 to 138 mg/dl. Heparin was restarted and the EACA stopped. Over a nine day course of heparin the PT, PTT, platelets and fibrinogen returned towards normal and the skin lesions cleared.

Comment: This patient with Laennec's cirrhosis developed probable gram negative septicemia and DIC with fibrinolysis. Coagulation tests improved on heparin, and heparin and EACA, but deteriorated when EACA was given alone.

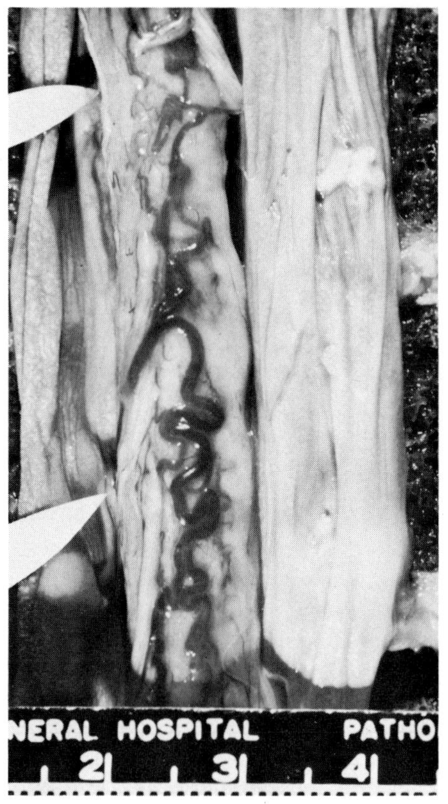

Figure XI–3. Thrombosed anterior median spinal artery in Figure XI–2.

NO HEPARIN OR EACA THERAPY

Patients who receive neither heparin nor EACA can improve completely (Tables XI-III and IV). In three instances the underlying disease process was promptly corrected, and with the stimulus for DIC gone, the coagulation abnormalities promptly disappeared (*see* histories of Case 19 in Chap. IV, and Case 30 in Chap. VI).

In contrast two thirds of the patients receiving neither heparin nor EACA, had underlying disease processes that could not be eradicated, and their bleeding and DIC worsened (*see* history of Case 4 in Chap. XIII) (Tables XI-III and IV).

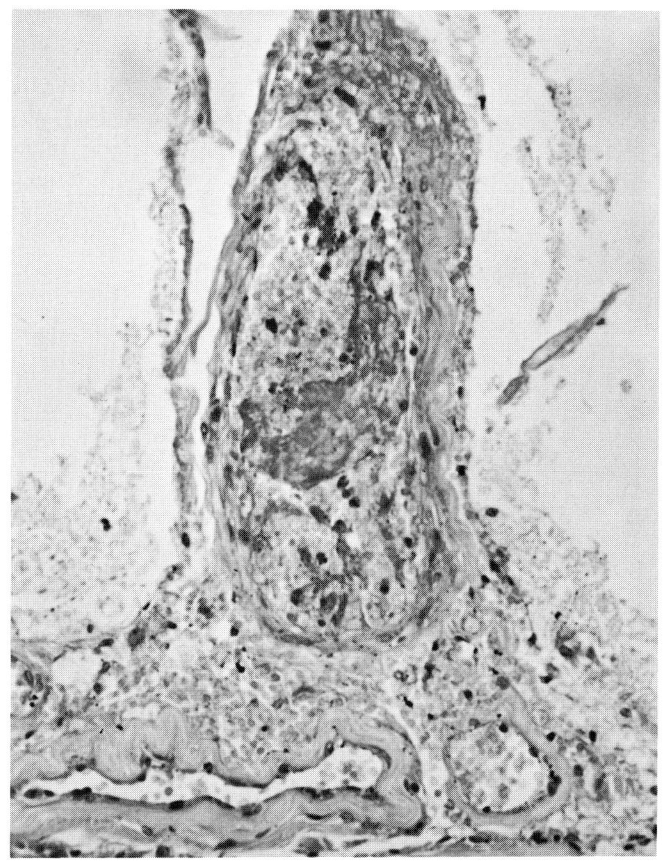

Figure XI–4. Cross section of Figure XI–3 showing fibrin thrombus in central branches of anterior median spinal artery. EACA was given for "primary fibrinolysis". (Hematoxylin and eosin stain, × 240.) (*Ibid.*)

COMPARISON OF HEPARINIZED AND NON-HEPARINIZED PATIENTS

No randomized trial of heparin therapy for DIC has yet been reported and our patients were *not* randomized into treatment groups. Despite this shortcoming, it is of interest to compare patients treated with heparin alone (in addition to primary disease therapy) with those receiving only therapy for their underlying diseases.

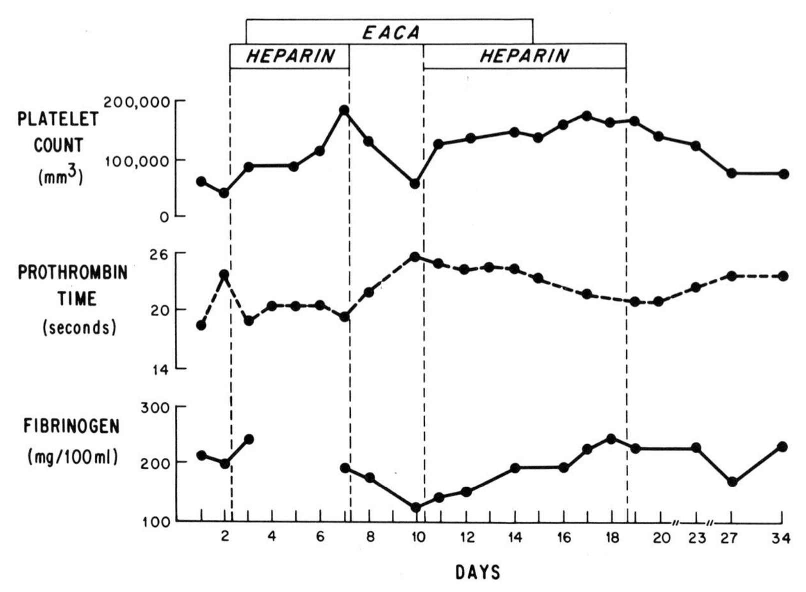

Figure XI–5. Case 10.

The groups were similar in age, sex, severity of bleeding, and incidence of hypotension. With the exception of FDP titers, there were no significant differences in coagulation tests at the time of diagnosis of DIC. Significant differences in primary disease were apparent: there was more septicemic DIC in the heparinized patients and more carcinoma-leukemia induced DIC in the nonheparinized group. The bleeding response was significantly better in the heparinized patients (Table XI-V). While the acute survival (ability to leave the hospital) of symptomatic patients was twice as great in the heparinized group, it was not statistically significant because of the small number of patients.

SUBCLINICAL DIC

A recurrent question is whether patients with subclinical DIC should be treated. Clinical signs such as the sudden appearance of hypotension in a patient with either suspected sepsis or isolated coagulation abnormalities suggest that the full syndrome of DIC is imminent. Rapid diagnosis is essential

TABLE XI-V
COMPARISON OF HEPARIN VERSUS NON-HEPARINIZED PATIENTS[1]

	Characteristics of Treatment Groups		
	Heparinized	Non-Heparinized	Significant Differences[2]
Number of patients	26	15	
Age, Years (mean)	46	43	−
Sex (% males)	58	40	−
Hypotension (%)	54	47	−
Etiology			
Septicemic (%)	69	27	+
Neoplastic (%)	23	40	+
Coagulation Tests[4]			
Before Therapy			
Prothrombin time (sec)	25	21	−
Platelets/μl	50	51	−
Fibrinogen (mg/dl)	132	118	−
Fi (titer $\log_2$)	7.5	4.8	+
After Therapy			
Prothrombin time (sec)	16	16	−
Platelets/μl	111,000	90,000	−
Fibrinogen (mg/dl)	299	195	+
Diminished Bleeding (%)	68	31	+[3]
Survival (%)			
All patients	38	33	−
Bleeding patients	37	17	−

[1] All patients included regardless of length of survival.
[2] + = $P < 0.05$.
[3] Statistically significant by X^2 analysis for the following response groups of heparinized vs. non-heparinized patients: complete improvement vs. bleeding worse $P < 0.001$; complete improvement vs. worse or indeterminant, $P < 0.05$; any improvement vs. worse or indeterminant, $P < 0.02$.
[4] In addition, no differences in ELT or TT were noted.

and one can argue that heparin therapy should be begun.

In contrast, patients in whom life threatening clinical signs are not expected to develop should probably not be treated. In the following example appropriate laboratory tests were performed as a teaching exercise to show that subclinical DIC can occur that is probably of little clinical import.

Case 11—Gonococcemia and subclinical DIC: A 21-year-old woman entered with painful ankles and knees of six days' duration. Examination revealed several palpable, slightly tender, 2–5 mm nodules on the left forearm and a single 5 mm erythematous macule on the anterior left calf. The left ankle was exquisitely tender, swollen and red. Both knees were mildly tender.

The hematocrit was 44%, WBC 12,800 with 82% neutrophils, PT and PTT normal, platelets 214,000/ul, and Fi 1:16. Cultures of the fluid from the left ankle grew out *N. gonorrhoeae*. Biopsy of the calf lesion disclosed marked perivascular lymphocytes and rare neutrophils in the papillary and reticular dermis. Several small veins contained fibrin thrombi (Fig. X–21). Penicillin therapy was given and she was discharged two weeks later.

Comment: This patient is presented as a case of subclinical DIC with gonococcemia. The presence of fibrin thrombi in the skin biopsy and a positive Fi titer establish that intravascular coagulation had occurred.

DISCUSSION

Therapy of DIC must be placed within a broader scheme of therapy of the patient, which includes treatment of basic underlying diseases and additional complicating conditions. A vigorous attack on the underlying disease process(es) which initiated the DIC must be undertaken. Correction of hypotension, volume deficits, hypoxemia, acidosis, sepsis, and administration of appropriate pressor agents are crucial in the therapy of DIC. In several instances only the underlying disease was treated and the outcome was successful. In contrast, many patients with uncontrolled, recrudescent or new underlying disease, redeveloped or continued to exhibit DIC. It is imperative to reinvestigate control of the underlying disease(s) when any deterioration in coagulation studies occurs; similarly, control of DIC should be reexamined if new disease processes develop.

In our patients, cessation of all major bleeding occurred in 79 percent of the patients treated with heparin in addition to therapy for the underlying disease(s). This result agrees with the experience of others (1,50,115,130). While reversal of the underlying disease processes is desirable, many (13 of 19) heparin-treated patients showed significant improvement in bleeding status and coagulation studies despite unchanged underlying diseases. Although initial clinical examination did not indicate those patients who would respond to therapy, coagulation tests at the time of diagnosis and after therapy were well correlated with clinical response. Within an average of three days, the patients whose bleeding eventually stopped showed normalization of the PT, high levels of fibrinogen (average 314 mg/dl) but a variable rise in platelet count. In the group with continued bleeding, the PT rose, the platelets fell, and although the fibrinogen level rose, the increment was significantly less than in the improved group (Table X-II).

These data suggest that nearly normal values for PT and high levels of fibrinogen have to be achieved for improvement to occur. In contrast, the lack of an immediate platelet response is not necessarily a bad prognostic sign; in many cases the platelet count did not rise for ten to fourteen days, a finding noted also by others (38,116). Bone marrow depression and myelophthisis are important factors governing the platelet response.

The time in which the FDP titer falls is variable. The Fi titer fell to normal in hours in some cases, but when the titer was markedly elevated resolution took over a week to occur.

The frequent occurrence of increased bleeding shortly after initiation of heparin therapy raised the question of whether heparin can exaggerate bleeding in a patient whose hemostatic system is already severely compromised. If a patient without DIC or other hemostatic abnormalities is placed on heparin, the incidence of bleeding will be about 7 percent (160); this is in contrast to the 85 percent of patients with DIC who are bleeding before therapy and 60 percent of whom will show transitorily increased bleeding shortly after heparin is administered. The coagulation data at the time of increased bleeding suggested that this was related to DIC rather than to heparin.

If the PT, platelets and fibrinogen levels are worse or unchanged, we feel heparin therapy should be maintained or increased as a high percentage of these patients will subsequently stop bleeding. Any sign of bleeding into the pulmonary or central nervous system warrants careful evaluation of the hemostatic state. Only one patient (Case 17) had a serious complication possibly due to heparin therapy; however, other factors unrelated to DIC could not be excluded. Thus heparin therapy appears relatively safe in the presence of DIC with a bleeding diathesis. Other reported, but rare complications of heparin during short term therapy are hypersensitivity reaction, alopecia, and acute reversible thrombocytopenia (72,144).

The choice of heparin dosage depends on coagulation test response, bleeding status, and the underlying disease state. We usually begin with 70–80 USP units/kg in adult patients administered intravenously every four hours. Knowing the level of fibrinogen associated with cessation of bleeding (> 300 mg/dl) and the dose response curve for heparin (Fig. XI-1), the dose of heparin can be increased until the appropriate response is obtained. If bleeding persists and the appropriate coagulation test response is not achieved over a three to four day period (the time normally required for a response) the dose may be increased by small increments and a thorough reevaluation of the underlying disease processes made.

It seems reasonable that heparin therapy be maintained as long as the acute underlying disease process is active (approximately 3–7 days in our patients). When heparin is discontinued the coagulation tests should be monitored for deterioration. The heparin therapy was nearly always discontinued abruptly in our patients, but gradual tapering of dosage might be advisable when a chronic precipitating condition such as neoplasia is present.

Heparin is metabolized in the liver to an inactive form which is then excreted by the kidney (73). Liver failure may require a reduction in dosage. However, patients with liver disease and patients with azotemia have received standard doses without complication.

Review of the literature suggests that heparin therapy may be valuable in treating the DIC that is secondary to a wide variety of diseases.

Infectious diseases are among the most frequent causes of DIC, accounting for 40 percent of our patients. One of the classic associations is fulminant meningococcemia. Both favorable responses to heparin (112,216) and lack of effect on clinical outcome (38,48) have been reported.

That DIC occurs in other types of gram negative sepsis has only recently been recognized. Few cases have been treated with heparin. In the only large series reported, Corrigan and Jordan (38) concluded that heparin does not improve survival in patients with septicemia and hypotension. However, many patients died within 24 hours of initiation of heparin therapy, which their own data suggests is too short of a period in which to expect improvement.

DIC occurs commonly in viral infections (118), especially the exanthematous diseases, including varicella, variola, rubella and rubeola, and in arbor viruses. It occurs also with other viral diseases, such as cytomegalic inclusion disease (93). Virtually all the hemorrhagic fevers, including Thai, Bolivian, Argentine and Philippine, implicate DIC as the most important mechanism of bleeding. In a non-randomized study of the effectiveness of heparin in Philippine hemorrhagic fever (118), bleeding stopped sooner, platelet and fibrinogen levels recovered more rapidly and survival was higher in heparin treated patients.

Instances of successful treatment of DIC with heparin have been reported in malaria (41), and scrub typhus (24). Another cause of DIC is the post-infectious sequela, purpura fulminans. Survival in this disease was rare prior to the use of heparin (106).

Chronic DIC that occurs with carcinoma affords the possibility of using the patient as his own control. Thus, in a patient with metastic carcinoma of the prostate with DIC (194) manifested by hemorrhage, hypofibrinogenemia, thrombocytopenia, and fibrinolysis (long TT, rapid ELT and elevated FDP), heparin abolished on four separate occasions all evidence of the fibrinolysis.

Mosesson *et al.* (135) reported a case of DIC characterized by transient cerebral ischemic attacks associated with a low fibrinogen, low platelets and cryofibrinogenemia. A carcinoma of the ovary was eventually discovered. After heparin treatment, the platelets and fibrinogen rose and the cryofibrinogenemia decreased; on stopping heparin these changes reversed and cerebro-vascular thrombosis ensued. The patient remained on heparin for eighteen months without thrombotic or hemorrhagic complications.

Other types of carcinoma where DIC responded to heparin included colon (130), lung (87), stomach (207) and pancreas (71). DIC has been successfully treated in leukemia of the stem cell (52), myelocytic (6) and promyelocytic (208) varieties.

Intrauterine fetal death is another example of chronic

intravascular coagulation in which heparin has favorably altered a situation where failure of hemostasis frequently occurs. The clinical picture is gradual depletion of fibrinogen and other coagulation factors along with the appearance of cryofibrinogen (7) and FDP (65), probably due to release of thromboplastic substances derived from placental and fetal autolysis. This syndrome may lead only to a mild hemorrhagic tendency. Then in association with delivery or some other surgical or traumatic event, severe bleeding ensues.

If severe bleeding has already ensued, rapid evacuation of the uterus is indicated. In several cases (7,65) heparin has reversed the coagulation abnormalities with a rise in fibrinogen, platelets and other clotting factors with a fall in cryofibrinogen and FDP. The improvement allowed safe surgical termination of pregnancy without the potential hazards of fibrinogen or transfusions. Heparin is usually stopped shortly before surgical evacuation of the uterus.

The chronic intravascular coagulation must be distinguished from the acute DIC of abruptio placentae, in which pregnancy must be terminated rapidly. Heparin therapy may have no place in this self-limited acute problem, although together with replacement therapy (whole blood and fibrinogen) it has been used in seven of eight cases with good results (207).

Despite numerous reports about the efficacy of heparin, dissenting views have been expressed. No randomized study has ever been performed, and undoubtedly one would be extremely difficult to carry out. Although our patients were not randomized into treatment groups, they received similar treatment for their underlying diseases within the same hospital and were observed using the same criteria for diagnosis and evaluation of response to therapy.

Significant differences in favor of heparin therapy were found for bleeding response and improvement in fibrinogen level. Significant differences were not detected for response of prothrombin time, platelet count or overall survival. However, the heparin-treated group did have twice as great a surviving fraction as the non-heparinized patients. The groups were well-matched in most respects, but major differences in primary diseases existed between them: there was more septicemia and less neoplasia in the heparinized patients.

To obtain information of the influence of heparin on survival in DIC, a single causative disease group was selected in which sufficient numbers of patients were available for statistical analysis. The data on survival in septicemic patients with DIC from our series (prospective and retrospective) were pooled with that of Corrigan and Jordan (38) (pediatric patients), Najjar and Ahmad (142) (pediatric patients) and Yoshikawa *et al.* (221) (largely patients with septic abortions). It should be noted that pediatric and septic obstetrical problems dominated these series.

If all patients were compared without regard to length of survival, the percent survival is greater in the heparin-treated group, but not at a statistically significant level (Table XI-VI). Because our data indicated that regardless of therapy a significant length of time elapsed before a bleeding response was obtained, it appeared instructive to examine those patients who survived for more than a few hours after diagnosis of DIC.

When patients surviving for more than one day in the

TABLE XI-VI
SURVIVAL IN SEPTICEMIC DIC[1]
(Number of Patients)

All Patients Regardless of Lengths of Survival

Therapy	Survive	Die	Total	% Survive	X^2	P
Heparin	24	35	59	41	3.114	< 0.1
None	6	22	28	21		
TOTAL	30	57	87	35%		

Ultimate Survival in Patients Living > 24 Hours

Therapy	Survive	Die	Total	% Survive	X^2	P
Heparin	24	12	36	67	6.175	< 0.025
None	6	13	19	32		
TOTAL	30	25	55	55%		

[1] Pooled data from present study (patients 1–45, i-xv), Corrigan and Jordan (38), Najjar and Ahmad (142), and from the references cited in Yoshikawa *et al.* (221).

untreated group are compared to the heparin-treated group, there is significantly increased survival of the patients receiving heparin. While the pathophysiology and treatment of those patients dying with fulminating septicemia and DIC remains to be elucidated, our data and analysis of other series suggests heparin probably is of therapeutic importance (37).

Patients receiving EACA alone showed either clinical or laboratory deterioration, confirming other reports (23,76,119). Although there is insufficient data from our study to indicate whether heparin or heparin/EACA therapy is superior, our data and other reports (194) indicate that heparin alone is sufficient to abolish fibrinolysis (*see* "Systemic Fibrinolysis", Chap. VI).

More important is the finding that fibrinolysis without DIC is rare as first noted by Merskey *et al* (130), and because of this the therapeutic dilemma of heparin vs EACA is in practice not a problem. We agree with previous investigators (168) that all fibrinolysis be assumed to be secondary to DIC and that heparin should be instituted before EACA therapy is started.

DIC can increase in severity when fibrinogen is administered without concurrent heparin therapy (82). Although several patients in the series received heparin and fibrinogen, fibrinogen concentrates appear unnecessary because of the rapidity with which the body produces fibrinogen under stress (217) and also because of the risk of hepatitis. As a useful approximation, one unit of plasma or blood should raise the plasma fibrinogen by 25 mg/dl in a 70 kg individual. In addition, the prothrombin complex factors and factors V and VIII will be corrected by fresh frozen plasma. This would seem to be the best choice for factor replacement in the severely bleeding patient after the red cell requirement has been met. Often coagulation studies are obtained after transfusion; under these conditions borderline low fibrinogen values become even more significant. Recently cryoprecipitates have been used to supply fibrinogen and factor VIII; however, they lack factor V.

Platelet administration may lead to the development of isoantibodies; most patients who improved did not receive platelet concentrates. Only in those patients who are bleeding severely or bleeding into critical sites might a vigorous course of fresh frozen plasma and platelet concentrates be attempted after heparin therapy was started.

There should be some optimism concerning the outcome of DIC. Half of patients stopped bleeding completely and 74 percent showed cessation of all major bleeding. One fourth of the patients with bleeding and hypotension (8/33) survived to leave the hospital. While the mortality rate of the patients who bled most severely was 100 percent, a large proportion survived for greater than four days after the onset of DIC, indicating that there should be time to institute therapy against the underlying disease.

CHAPTER XII

VALIDATION OF CRITERIA FOR DIAGNOSIS OF DIC—RETROSPECTIVE ANALYSIS

SCREENING CRITERIA

SINCE NO ONE TEST IS AS YET accepted as pathognomonic of DIC, the problem of validation of diagnostic criteria arises. The triad of simultaneously occuring prolonged PT, thrombocytopenia, and hypofibrinogenemia suggests DIC, and is found in many of the literature reports. This group of tests has formed the clinical basis for our diagnostic scheme. Figure XII-1 and Table XII-I show the evaluation of 91 patients we examined for consideration of DIC (45 patients included in the prospective study and 46 patients initially excluded whose case histories were evaluated retrospectively).

The coagulation criteria separate patients into clinically distinct groups with respect to symptoms and underlying diseases. Thirty-five of the 91 patients met the 3/3 screening criteria. Thirty-one (87%) had positive tests of fibrinolysis. Of four of 36 patients whose Fi, ELT or TT were negative, we were able to follow only one in the prospective series (Case 27), and this patient had an abnormal TRCHII indicating presence of FDP. Retrospective examination of the other three case histories (Table XII-II, Cases i-iii) disclosed that all had bleeding and clinical settings suggestive of DIC. Their Fi titers were within the normal range (1:4 – 1:8).

The 56 patients with less than three abnormal screening tests posed the major diagnostic problem. For these patients, the presence of fibrinolysis was demanded as an additional diagnostic criteria. The data show internal agreement; patients meeting 2/3 criteria with positive tests of fibrinolysis

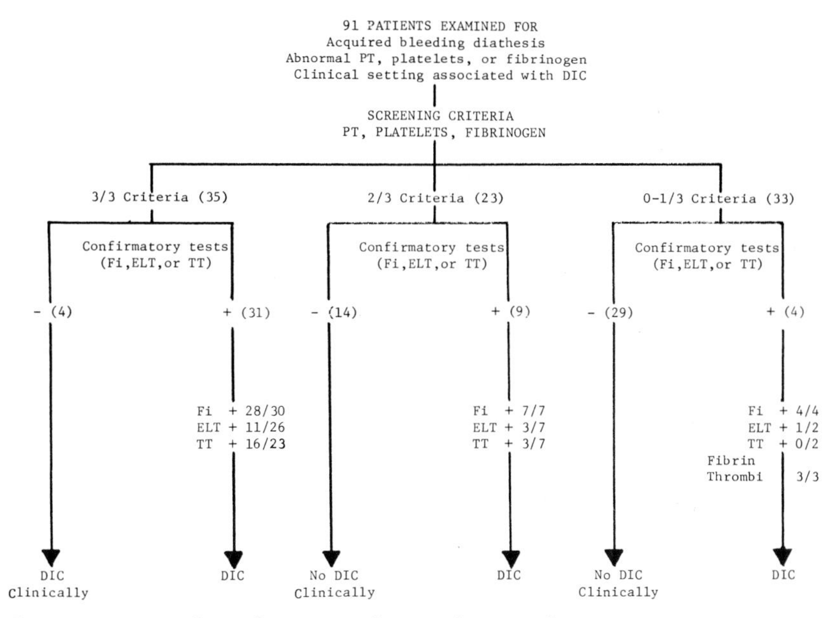

Figure XII–1. Flow diagram of coagulation changes in 91 patients screened for DIC. *Screening criteria* are given in Tables I-I and II. Numbers in parentheses represent number of patients. *DIC Clinically* represents documentation of fibrin thrombi, and/or multisite bleeding associated with septicemia, neoplasia, and/or hypotension.

had clinical settings consistent with DIC (hypotension, sepsis, or neoplasia) and nearly always bleeding or thrombosis.

In a retrospective review of the clinical histories and pathological materials of the group meeting the 2/3 criteria, but in whom the tests for fibrinolysis were negative, few patients had bleeding or illnesses typically associated with DIC; no patient had fibrin thrombi at autopsy; these patients were often referred primarily for PT or platelet count abnormalities, but not once for hypofibrinogenemia.

Four patients met the 0–1/3 screening criteria with FDP and fibrin thrombi and are included as examples of DIC with minimal laboratory derangement. Two of these patients (Cases 15,31) had severe thrombotic or acral cyanotic episodes. None of the 29 patients meeting one or less of the screening criteria and having no FDP had bleeding, thrombi or acrocyanosis.

TABLE XII-I
COMPARISON OF CLINICAL STATUS AND COAGULATION TESTS IN PATIENTS INCLUDED OR EXCLUDED FROM STUDY[1]

	Criteria met (N = 48)	Criteria not met (N = 43)
Diagnostic criteria used:		
3/3 Screening tests abnormal	35	0
& tests of fibrinolysis positive	32	
& tests of fibrinolysis negative	3	
2/3 Sreening tests abnormal		
& tests of fibrinolysis positive	9	0
0–1/3 Screening tests abnormal		
& tests of fibrinolysis positive	4	0
Fibrin thrombi	22/30	0/4
PT >15 sec	90%	49%
Platelets <150,000/μl	94%	4%
Fibrinogen <160 mg/dl	73%	0%
Fibrinogen >410 mg/dl	0%	40%
Bleeding	88%	30%
Thrombosis-acral cyanosis	23%	0%
Survival	33%	57%
DIC terminated by time of consultation	3/48[2]	0/43

[1] Comparison of all data significant (Chi square) at $p < 0.001$, except "survival" where $p < 0.05$.
[2] Patients i, ii, iii, Table XII-II.

SPECIFICITY OF HYPOFIBRINOGENEMIA IN THE DIAGNOSIS OF DIC

Many causes for prolonged PT and thrombocytopenia exist but the causes of hypofibrinogenemia are few. In reviewing all fibrinogen determinations performed by the MGH clinical chemistry laboratory from November 1967 through June 1969, 13 percent of 860 patients had fibrinogen levels below 160 mg/dl (i.e., more than two standard deviations from the norm). Twenty-six of these patients (24%) were included in our study. Review of the available case histories and pathologic materials of the remaining patients revealed that these patients fell into three distinct groups: (a) DIC (Cases i-xv, Table XII-II) (49%); (b) severe liver disease (17%); or (c) were on cardiopulmonary bypass (34%). There were no cases of unexplained hypofibrinogenemia.

A histogram of all in-patient fibrinogen determinations reveals a bimodal distribution (Fig. XII-2). The lower peak agrees with the mean established for normals (247 vs 230 mg/dl). The higher of the two peaks was similar to the levels in our patients prior to the onset of DIC (368 vs 365 mg/dl). It is known that fibrinogen levels are elevated in inflammatory conditions and in acutely ill patients (217). Thus, the patients with a prolonged PT and thrombocytopenia, but with fibrinogen levels within a normal range (2/3 screening criteria) appear to have "relative hypofibrinogenemia." Prior to DIC their average fibrinogen is elevated (532 mg/dl), while during DIC their mean fibrinogen level falls to 243 mg/dl and after therapy their average fibrinogen level rises to 391 mg/dl (Table I-III).

EFFECT OF HYPOFIBRINOGENEMIA ON TESTS OF COAGULATION

In congenital hypofibrinogenemia, the fibrinogen level must fall below 55 mg/dl to prolong the PT by three seconds (83,218), while the fibrinogen concentration has to fall below 75 mg/dl before the TT becomes prolonged by five seconds (definition of an abnormal TT in DIC). Analysis of the patient data confirms this: all patients with fibrinogen levels below 75 mg/dl have abnormal thrombin times (Table XII-III). Thus, the TT can only be used for diagnosis of fibrinolysis when the fibrinogen level is above 75 mg/dl. When the fibrinogen was higher, half of the TTs were still abnormal. This probably reflects the anticoagulant effect of circulating FDP (36,96). Since the TT can detect both circulating FDP and severe hypofibrinogenemia, it is useful diagnostically when abnormal.

The relationship of ELT to fibrinogen level is complex and depends on the plasminogen:fibrinogen ratio used in forming the clot (129). The ELT in plasmin-rich clots is independent of the clot fibrin concentration (129). Analysis of our patient data showed no significant correlation between ELT and fibrinogen level (Table XII-III).

SIGNIFICANCE OF FIBRIN THROMBI

Because of the small number of fibrin thrombi sometimes demonstrated histologically in cases of DIC, the specificity

TABLE XII-II
15 ADDITIONAL CASES OF DIC FOUND IN A RETROSPECTIVE STUDY OF HYPOFIBRINOGENEMIA

Case	Clinical Diagnosis from Hospital Record	PT (sec)	Platelet (per μl)	Fibrinogen (mg/dl)	Bleeding	Survival	Comment
i	Homocystinuria Bronchopneumonia, DIC	15	34,000	30	+	–	Fi 1:8
ii	Klebsiella Septicemia, DIC	16	38,000	90	+	–	Fi 1:8
iii	Septic Abortion β Streptococcal septicemia	18	12,000	120	+	–	Fi 1:4
iv	Pseudomonas septicemia, DIC	25	49,000	90	+	–	
v	Bronchogenic carcinoma widely metastatic, DIC	17	68,000	120	+	–	
vi	Lymphoblastic lymphoma Herpes zoster, Thrombophlebitis	16	76,000	90	+	–	Chlorambucil and Prednisone
vii	Acute myelomonocytic leukemia	19	17,000	132	+	+	6-Mercaptopurine & cytosine arabinoside
viii	Pregnancy (stillborn) Acute pancreatitis, DIC	22	44,000	40	+	+	
ix	Klebsiella pneumonia	18	152,000	110	+	+	
x	Biliary atresia, Post op *S. albus* septicemia & peritonitis	27	78,000	102	+	–	
xi	Hodgkin's disease	17	23,000	130	+	–	Vincristine & Nitrogen must.
xii	Post op resection gastric ulcer Aspiration pneumonitis Thrombophlebitis and Pulmonary emboli massive	18	55,000	60	+	–	

xiii	*P. falciparum* malaria, DIC	22	15,000	160	+	+	Fi test 1:16
xiv	Laennec's cirrhosis, Gastritis, DIC	28	46,000	48	+	–	
xv	Idiopathic thrombocytopenic purpura[1]	15	10,000	130	+	+	Retic 15% Post splenectomy Serum hemoglobin 22 mg/dl (DIC 2° hemolysis)
	Average Values, Patients i-xv	18	57,000	108[2]			
	Average Values, Patients 1–45	18	52,000	137			

[1] Probable DIC

[2] Preselection for hypofibrinogenimia explains why the mean fibrinogen value is lower in patients i-xv than in patients 1-45.

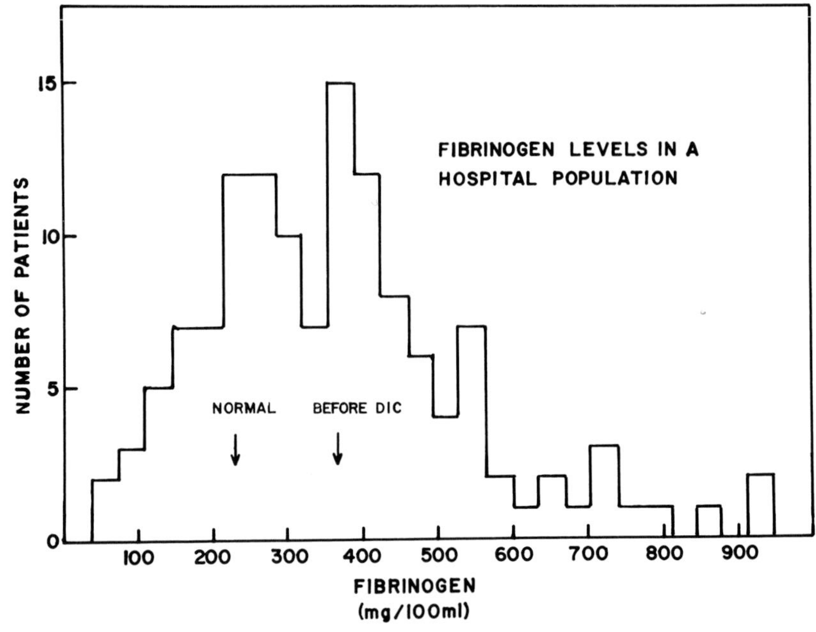

Figure XII–2. Histogram of all fibrinogen levels performed on hospitalized patients by MGH Clinical Chemistry Laboratory (four month period). The lowest value was selected when multiple determinations were performed. The arrows indicate the mean values for 17 personnel in our laboratory (normal), and 23 patients in this study who subsequently developed DIC. Note the correspondence of the two peaks with the arrows.

TABLE XII-III
EFFECT OF FIBRINOGEN CONCENTRATION IN PATIENT PLASMA ON THROMBIN TIME AND EUGLOBULIN CLOT LYSIS TIME

		FIBRINOGEN mg/dl			
		< 75		> 75	
THROMBIN TIME	ABNORMAL	8		11	$P < 0.025$
	NORMAL	0		12	
		< 100	100–160	> 160	
EUGLOBULIN CLOT LYSIS TIME	ABNORMAL	9	2	5	*P* not significant
	NORMAL	9	8	6	

of finding a single fibrin thrombus was examined (Table XII-IV). Kidney histology was reviewed in 300 consecutive autopsies performed by the MGH Pathology Department from November 1967 through January 1968. One or more fibrin thrombi were found in 7.3 percent of the cases. Only one of these patients was included in the present series.

Review of the case histories and autopsy protocols indicated that at least 64 percent of these patients probably had DIC (evidenced by bleeding diathesis, septicemia, shock, or abnormal coagulation data). Most of these patients entered the hospital only hours to a day before death, which explains why the DIC or infection was not suspected clinically or could not be documented premortem. The remaining 36 percent of patients probably had renal emboli (cardiac surgery, valvular, or aortic vessel disease), although some also had settings for DIC (cardiac arrest or prolonged hypotension). Coagulation studies were performed in only a few patients; all were abnormal or changing in the direction postulated by DIC. This data suggests that the presence of even a single well-formed thrombus in the absence of an embolic source is evidence in favor of the diagnosis of DIC. Others have reached similar conclusions (139).

TABLE XII-IV

ANALYSIS OF FIBRIN THROMBI IN 300 CONSECUTIVE AUTOPSIES

Etiology of Fibrin Thrombi	# Patients		Frequency
DIC, probable	9		64%
Septicemia		6	
Metastatic carcinoma		2	
Lymphoma, chemotherapy		1	
Embolic[1]			
(Heart valve replacement, aortic aneurysm resection, aortic mural thrombi)	5		36%

[1] Four of the five patients also had settings for DIC (prolonged hypotension or cardiac arrest).

CHAPTER XIII

LIVER DISEASE IN DIC

DIAGNOSIS AND THERAPY IN THE bleeding patient with liver disease poses special problems. In uncomplicated cirrhosis the coagulation and fibrinolytic tests may be abnormal, even though no clinically significant hemostatic defects (e.g., DIC) are present (46,198). The damaged liver is compromised in two functions essential to the maintenance of normal hemostasis: synthesis of coagulation proteins and clearance of activated procoagulants and fibrinolytic activators.

The liver normally synthesizes fibrinogen, factor V and factor XIII. A second synthetic system which is dependent on vitamin K, produces the prothrombin complex composed of factor II, VII, IX and X. In the steady state the rate of synthesis is equal to the rate of degradation. When synthesis of these proteins is decreased in liver disease, factor VII may become limiting since it has the shortest half life of any coagulation protein, five to six hours (101). Since the PT is extremely sensitive to factor VII concentrations (*see* "PT" in Chapter II), this clotting test is frequently abnormal in liver disease.

Perhaps equally central to the pathogenesis of bleeding disorders in liver disease is defective clearance of activated enzymes and coagulation factors. It is currently believed that hepatocellular enzymes inactivate activated factors IX, X, and XI (188). In contrast large molecules, including prothrombinase, a lipid-protein complex, fibrin polymers and thromboplastin are cleared by the reticuloendothelial system which is primarily located in the liver. The liver also removes activators of plasminogen (61,153).

The blood flow to the liver, which may be disturbed either by damage to the portal vein or by intrinsic disease to the liver itself, is critical in maintaining a normal hemostatic homeostasis. For example, when factor X in a presursor state is injected intravenously into a normal person the half life is 40 hours (42). After it is activated it is cleared within minutes (42). During the brief time this activated protein circulates systemically, a true hypercoagulable state results. During the short period of hypercoagulability, blood will rapidly clot if the circulation stops (211,212). If the activated factor X is infused into the portal vein rather than into the systemic circulation, the length of the hypercoagulable state is greatly decreased. Conversely, if the activated coagulant is blocked from entering the hepatic circulation, the true hypercoagulable state remains and DIC ensues (211).

The cirrhotic liver is a compromised organ that behaves as if part of its circulation were occluded. The cirrhotic liver requires ten times longer than the normal organ to clear activated plasminogen (61). The result of the impaired clearing function is to lower greatly the defenses of the cirrhotic patient to the effects of activated coagulation factors or an activated fibrinolytic system.

Patients with cirrhosis, who are stable, not bleeding, and not under stress, e.g., without superimposed infection, appear to be in a state of compensated DIC. In a study by Tytgat (197) fifty patients with documented cirrhosis were compared to normal subjects. The fibrinogen concentrations of the two populations were not significantly different. However the half survival time of the fibrinogen in cirrhotic patients was one day shorter (3 vs 4 days) than normal patients, indicating that the catabolic rate of fibrinogen in cirrhosis was increased by about a third. This increased rate could be secondary to increased fibrinogen conversion to fibrin by thrombin or increased digestion by activated fibrinolysins. Although heparin therapy resulted in the catabolic rate returning to normal and a rise in fibrinogen levels, treatment with fibrinolytic inhibitors had no effect. These data indicated that subclinical DIC probably occurs continuously in patients with cirrhosis. Using slightly different experimental techniques others have reached similar conclusions (17).

When a patient with liver disease bleeds, local causes (e.g. varices, ulcers), impaired synthesis of coagulation factors, thrombocytopenia secondary to hypersplenism, DIC and fibrinolysis are potential etiologies either singly or in combination. In addition a superimposed and unrelated disease, e.g., septicemia, must be considered (*see* history of Case 37 below).

CASE 37—LAENNEC'S CIRRHOSIS, HEPATIC ENCEPHALOPATHY, STREPTOCOCCAL SEPTICEMIA, AND GENERALIZED BLEEDING: A 60 year-old man with Laennec's cirrhosis entered in impending hepatic coma precipitated by dental surgery. One year previously, a portacaval shunt and splenectomy were performed because of bleeding esophageal varices; the PT at that time was 22 sec, platelet count 116,000/ul and fibrinogen 160 mg/dl.

By the second hospital day the encephalopathy was worse, mucosal bleeding began and purpura appeared on the flank. The PT was 25 sec, platelet count 91,000/ul, fibrinogen 80 mg/dl, ELT 55 minutes, Fi 1:64, and SCT 1:128. The kallikrein system was markedly activated (Table VIII-III). Multiple blood cultures grew out streptococcus, Group D.

Heparin (6200 units every 4 hr) and penicillin were begun. One day later the bleeding was more brisk and was present in the nasogastric aspirate, stools, oral-nasal mucosa, urine (gross blood), venipuncture sites, traumatic lesion on the scalp, and as xanthochromia in spinal fluid.

Because the clotting time remained normal, the dosage of heparin was raised to 9400 units (every 4 hr). During the next three days the bleeding slowed markedly, the ELT returned to normal, the Fi titer fell from 1:64 to 1:16 (Fig. VI-2). The PT fell to baseline levels, while the platelet count remained at abnormally low levels for the patient. The patient remained in coma and died on the sixth day. No autopsy was performed.

Comment: This case is an example of severe liver disease with superimposed septicemia. Chronically he had decreased synthesis of coagulation factors, mild thrombocytopenia, and varices as potential bleeding sites. Acutely he developed DIC as evidenced by the multisite bleeding and marked deterioration in coagulation factors. In this instance kallikrein determinations were of aid in assessing the significance of the septicemic process and hence a possible etiology for the DIC. The bleeding and coagulation abnormalities responded to heparin therapy.

The usual criteria for DIC (Table I-I) are not applicable to patients with liver disease since many would certainly be met even if the patient were in a stable state. In particular, tests for fibrinolysis would almost always be positive.

To approach this problem the criteria used must reflect a more severely deranged hemostatic system. We use criteria for diagnosis of DIC in liver disease that represent values more than two standard deviations from the mean in uncomplicated cirrhosis (Table XIII-I), or approximately three to four standard deviations outside the mean values for normal patients.

The clinical usefulness of these criteria is seen when they are applied to bleeding patients with liver disease (Table XIII-II). Comparison of the patients with liver disease meeting the criteria with those excluded showed the two groups to be distinct clinically. The rejected group had significantly more variceal bleeding, while the group with DIC bled from other sites. The group with DIC also had a higher incidence of septicemia, and a lower incidence of cirrhosis. Some of the patients meeting the criteria have received heparin therapy and all showed clinical and coagulation improvement.

TABLE XIII-I
CRITERIA FOR DIAGNOSIS OF DIC WHEN LIVER DISEASE IS PRESENT[1]

Test	Uncomplicated Cirrhosis[2] (Mean ± SD)	Abnormal Value for DIC (Criteria)	Mean Value DIC (9 Patients)[3]
Screening			
PT	14 ± 2 sec	>25 sec	29 sec
Platelets	176,000 ± 70,000/μl	<50,000/μl	35,000/μl
Fibrinogen	204 ± 55 mg/dl	<125 mg/dl	85 mg/dl
Confirmatory			
Fi Titer	≤1:16	≥1:32	1 : 84
TT	92% Abnormal	Not used	86%
ELT	67% Abnormal	Not used	57%

When liver disease is present the diagnosis of DIC requires:
1. 3 / 3 Screening Criteria for liver disease, or
2. Response to heparin therapy and meet regular criteria.

[1] Patients were considered as having liver disease if any of the following features were manifest: jaundice (bilirubin < 3 mg/dl); cirrhosis suspected clinically (portal hypertension or esophageal varices), histologically, or at laparotomy; recent hepatitis; or centrilobular congestion (serum lactic dehydrogenase (LDH) > 1000 units and glutamic oxalacetic transaminase (SGOT) > 800 Karmen units) due to congestive heart failure and confirmed by autopsy.

[2] Source of data: Prothrombin time, platelet count reference #46, fibrinogen level, Fi titer reference #198. The prothrombin time in reference #46 was expressed as the ratio of patient time to control time (average 1.16 ± 0.16). This was converted to seconds for the above comparison using 12 sec as a control time. The average fibrinogen level in reference # 46 was 316 ± 73 mg/dl. None of the 30 patients with chronic liver disease studied by Donaldson et al. (46) met any of the above screening criteria.

[3] Cases: 4, 6, 10, 33, 35, 37, 40, 45, xiv.

TABLE XIII-II

DIAGNOSIS OF DIC IN THE PRESENCE OF LIVER DISEASE[1]

	Patients meeting criteria[2]	Patients not meeting criteria	P value
Total. patients	9	9	
Mean coagulation values			
PT (sec)	29	19	
Platelets (/ul)	35,000	85,000	
Fibrinogen (mg/dl)	81	168	
Fi titer	1 : 84	1 : 12	
Clinical characteristics			
Bleeding	9	9	
Cirrhosis	4	9	<0.025
Variceal bleeding	2	8	<0.01
Non-variceal bleeding	8	5	<0.025
Septicemia	7	2	<0.01
Response to heparin	3 / 3	None treated	
Fibrin thrombi	6 / 7	0 / 1	
Mortality	8 / 9	7 / 9	

This analysis includes 18 patients. Eight patients are from the prospective study (Cases 4, 6, 10, 33, 35, 37, 40, 45); we examined each patient and all met the criteria set forth in Table XIII/I. An additional five patients were found in the group of 91 patients who were originally referred to us for possible DIC, but in whom we did not feel that DIC was present (*see* Chap I); these patients were personally examined and none met the coagulation criteria for DIC and liver disease. The last five patients are from the retrospective analysis of hypofibrinogenemia (*see* Chap. XIII); only one of these patients met the coagulation criteria (Table XII-II, case xiv); we examined none of these patients.

[2] Criteria, *see* Table XIII-I.

Six of seven patients with DIC and liver disease also had fibrin thrombi.

Thus the additional criteria demanded for the diagnosis of DIC when liver disease is present, appear to separate two clinically distinct classes of patients. In most of our patients some other pathological conditions, such as sepsis or hypotension, were superimposed on the liver disease and lead to the development of clinically significant DIC. The problems in diagnosis are well illustrated by the history of patient 10 (*see* "EACA Therapy" in Chap. XI), and patient 4 (*see* below).

CASE 4—CONGENITAL HEART DEFECTS, HEPATIC CONGESTION AND BLEEDING DIATHESIS: A three-day-old girl entered in respiratory distress. The pregnancy, delivery and first two days of life were unremarkable. The liver was rock hard and enlarged. Peripheral perfusion was good but the femoral pulses were not palpable. The hematocrit was 47%, WBC 15,750, pH 7.07, pO_2 65 mmHg, glucose 12 mg, BUN 22, and total bilirubin 6.1 mg with 2.0 mg/dl direct.

The cerebro-spinal fluid was slightly xanthochromic. Sodium bicarbonate, glucose, digitalis and antibiotics were given. Twelve hours after admission she vomited 4+ guaiac positive material and the hematocrit fell to 32%. The PT was 27 sec, platelets 24,000/ul, fibrinogen 96 mg/dl, Fi 1:20, TT 39 sec, and ELT normal. Vitamin K and transfusions of fresh blood were given.

On the second day, apneic spells, decorticate posturing, increasing hypoxia and hypotension developed. One day later generalized seizures began and repeat lumbar puncture yielded grossly bloody fluid. The bilirubin was 14 mg/dl and SGOT 2800 units. Over the next three days the liver slowly enlarged, the decorticate posturing persisted and the fibrinogen fell to 54 mg/dl. Death occurred on the seventh hospital day.

The autopsy showed congenital heart disease with a ventricular septal defect, coarctation of aorta and bicuspid aortic value; the liver showed marked centrilobular congestion with necrosis and fibrin thrombi. Hemorrhage into the lungs, gastrointestinal tract and brain was present.

Comment: This patient is an example of DIC associated with massive liver failure, severe acidosis and hypoxemia.

In another approach to the problem of the diagnosis of DIC in patients who have liver disease, Mokarhan *et al.* (134) examined 21 consecutive patients with Laennec's cirrhosis who were actively bleeding (from varices, gastritis, or ulcers); patients with superimposed septicemia were excluded. Because of the expected abnormalities of the PT, PTT, and TT, the following tests were used for the diagnosis of DIC and on this basis the patients were divided into two groups: decreasing platelet counts and fibrinogen levels, elevated FDP, and a positive serial dilution protamine sulfate test (note the criteria of Mokarhan *et al.* [134] were defined as changes in serial observations, whereas the criteria employed in Table XIII-I require only one observation).

Fourteen bleeding patients with no DIC had a mortality of only seven percent. The cause of death in the one patient was repeated episodes of hepatic encephalopathy that were unrelated to the episode of bleeding. In contrast the seven patients with DIC had a strikingly high mortality rate, 71 percent. In every case, hemorrhage was the major cause of death; 85 percent had evidence of ecchymosis and 71 percent, mucosal hemorrhage. The patients without DIC lacked mucosal bleeding and only 28 percent had ecchymosis. Hepatic coma and ascites were equally frequent in both groups, while the values for albumin, globulin, alkaline phosphatase, SGOT, SGPT, and total bilirubin were similar.

An important conclusion of Mokarhan *et al.*'s study (134) is that DIC can apparently occur with liver disease alone, or at least without obvious superimposed causes. It is apparent from the nature of the deaths in this group that generalized bleeding is an important factor leading to death. In contrast, their study also showed that patients with enhanced fibrinolysis and features of activated coagulation can compensate and recover spontaneously in some cases.

Summary

DIC can occur in patients with severe liver disease. For diagnosis, additional criteria (Table XIII-I) are needed beyond that normally used when liver disease is absent. When active bleeding occurs, DIC must be suspected on clinical grounds alone and superimposed factors such as septicemia or massive liver failure with acute hepatitis (166) should be sought. Regardless of etiology the presence of diffuse bleeding and coagulation criteria of DIC are indicative of serious disease in which the prognosis for survival is poor. In such a situation a trial of heparin seems indicated. Caution must be used in the dose chosen. Patients with liver dysfunctions show decreased metabolism of heparin and smaller doses are indicated in instituting therapy.

CHAPTER XIV

CLINICAL APPROACH TO A PATIENT WITH SUSPECTED DIC

GENERAL

ACQUIRED SEVERE HEMORRHAGIC diatheses are becoming an increasingly common situation in hospitals which care for critically ill patients. Meticulous attention to diagnostic and therapeutic detail are required if the patients are to survive. An approach to patients with suspected DIC is presented, followed by a discussion of certain complex but recurrent problems in management.

Tables XIV-I–XIV-III present a problem oriented clinical approach and Table X-VII an approach to the pathology of a patient suspected of having DIC. The approach includes ascertaining all conditions predisposing to DIC and other conditions affecting hemostasis, recognition of bleeding sites, anticipation of thrombotic complications, and estimation of response to therapy. A carefully taken and complete history, physical examination, and selection of appropriate laboratory tests including biopsy are essential. Repeated reexamination of the patient and careful quantification of response to therapy are also crucial.

In certain common clinical settings, DIC must be considered likely to appear. Thus signs of a developing hemorrhagic diathesis must be anticipated in patients with septicemia, obstetrical emergencies, cancer chemotherapy, acute promyelocytic leukemia, and shock. If hemorrhage appears or the patient is critically ill, screening coagulation tests (PT, platelets, fibrinogen) should be performed. Multisite bleeding, presence of thrombosis, acral cyanosis or necrotic skin lesions in the above settings should be regarded as highly suggestive of DIC. Finally, it is now commonplace

TABLE XIV-I

PROBLEM ORIENTED APPROACH TO A PATIENT WITH SUSPECTED DIC: HISTORY

Mode of presentation:
- Onset: Acute or chronic (of aid in identifying responsible underlying disease).
- Symptoms: Multi-site bleeding, thrombosis, acral cyanosis (recognition of an hemorrhagic diathesis).
- Disease Setting: Shock, septicemia, neoplasia (cancer chemotherapy), obstetric.
- Coagulation test abnormalities.

Underlying disease(s):
- Is more than one factor precipitating DIC?
- If no underlying disease is apparent, search for occult process.

Has DIC been previously documented?
- New disease precipitating DIC
- Recrudescence of old disease.
- Response to previous therapy.
  - Therapy of underlying diseases only.
  - Heparin: Dose, length of time.
  - EACA
  - Other: Vitamin K, folic acid, B_{12}, protamine, blood products, platelets, fibrinogen.

Search for other conditions affecting hemostasis:
- Hepatobiliary disease, malabsorption, uremia, anticoagulation, vitamin deficiency, marrow suppression, drug toxicity.

Symptoms of organ dysfunction:
- Life-threatening pulmonary or neurologic symptoms.
- Search for non-DIC related etiologies.

to screen seriously ill patients with a battery of diagnostic tests. Obviously, abnormalities of PT and platelet count that are unexplained suggest the possibility of DIC. Decreased fibrinogen is almost pathognomonic of DIC unless a past history of congenital afibrinogenemia or dysfibrinogenemia, L-asparaginase therapy, severe liver disease, or cardiopulmonary bypass is obtained.

All underlying disease(s) should be identified. If the clinical setting suggests DIC, one must carefully search for the various situations capable of precipitating DIC since correction of these factors is the first step in the successful therapy of DIC. Multiple etiologies in the individual patient are the rule rather than the exception. Thus hypotension, hypoxia, acidosis, septicemia, vascular injury by catheters, and liver damage should be specifically ruled out. If no underlying disease is apparent, occult processes such as intra-abdominal neoplasm or systemic fungal infection should be considered.

Has DIC been previously documented? The majority of patients who develop DIC will already be in the hospital,

TABLE XIV-II

PROBLEM ORIENTED APPROACH TO A PATIENT WITH SUSPECTED DIC: PHYSICAL EXAMINATION

- Bleeding:
  - Type: Multiple sites, local site, palpable purpura, massive subcutaneous hemorrhage, diffuse ooze, hematomas.
  - Severity
    - Direct observation: None, oozing, requiring transfusion, exsanguinating, severity of purpura (few, multiple, confluent).
    - Additional data: Calculation of fall in hematocrit, transfusion requirement, number of bleeding sites.
  - Location
    - Critical sites: Central nervous system, pulmonary (pulmonary hemorrhage syndrome), airway, pericardial. (Is pathological condition present in these sites that would predispose to bleeding?)
    - Specific areas: GI (upper, lower), GU, vaginal, pleural, tracheal-mucosal, fundus of eye, venipuncture, wound, injection sites, enteric catheters, venous-arterial cannulae.
- Thrombosis:
  - Large vessel or critical site
    - Neurologic examination: Does stroke syndrome exist?
    - Cardiovascular: Symptoms of pulmonary emboli?
    - Indwelling vascular catheter examination:
      - Does central venous pressure (CVP) catheter contain a thrombus?
      - Necrosis or gangrene impending in limbs with arterial cannulae?
  - Symptoms of impaired peripheral perfusion
    - Acral cyanosis (out of proportion to pO_2)
    - Documentation of pulses, capillary filling.
  - Diagnostic: Is a lesion accessible for biopsy?
  - Does a site for embolic development exist?
- Evaluation of organ and peripheral perfusion:
  - Blood pressure (postural hypotension), central venous pressure, urine output.
- Evaluation of underlying disease processes

and often they will have had one or more previous episodes of DIC. Much useful information can be gathered in this way. One should ask if, instead of the previous cause, a new unsuspected precipitating disease (such as occult sepsis) is responsible. Conversely, an old process can become recrudescent with the first manifestation being recurrent DIC. Present therapies (i.e. cancer chemotherapy) should be noted. Also previous therapies, such as vitamin K, folic acid, amount and type of blood products given should be considered. A unit of blood or plasma should theoretically increase the plasma fibrinogen by 25 mg/dl in a 70 kg individual. If multiple units of blood have been administered and the fibrinogen level is still low, concurrent consumption of fibrinogen is

TABLE XIV-III

PROBLEM ORIENTED APPROACH TO A PATIENT WITH SUSPECTED DIC: LABORATORY

Coagulation test abnormalities:
- Diagnostic triad: Prolonged prothrombin time, thrombocytopenia, hypofibrinogenemia
- Serial changes in coagulation tests.
  - Does relative hypofibrinogenemia exist?
- Relation of coagulation test abnormalities to symptoms, therapy, underlying disease.
- Evidence for fibrinolysis: Test for fibrinogen degradation products (Fi, staphylococcal clumping, tanned red cell hemagglutination inhibition), euglobulin clot lysis, thrombin time.

Peripheral blood smear and bone marrow:
- Schistocytosis (rarely of use)
- Evaluation of other causes of thrombocytopenia and anemia

Pathology
- Skin biopsy

Miscellaneous:
- Chest X-ray: Evidence of pulmonary hemorrhage syndrome?
- Body fluids: Search for other evidence of bleeding.
- Blood gas determination: Hypoxemia, acidosis?
- Blood culture: Undetected septicemia?
- Liver function: Additional criteria required for the diagnosis of DIC?

probable. If a patient has responded successfully to heparin therapy, the dose and time course of response are useful information in planning subsequent courses of therapy.

Other conditions affecting hemostasis should be excluded. A past and family history of bleeding should be obtained to rule out inherited bleeding tendencies, or chronic impairment of hemostasis. Drug toxicity affecting the bone marrow elements is extremely common. Likewise, ingestion of compounds that contain aspirin can impair platelet function. Administration of other anticoagulants, such as warfarin compounds, should be determined. Long term parenteral feedings can decrease folic acid and vitamin K intake and broad spectrum antibiotics can decrease folic acid absorption. The presence of hepatobiliary disease, malabsorption states and uremia are common sources of impaired hemostasis, either by diminished synthesis of coagulation factors, or impaired platelet function.

The principle types of organ dysfunction that appear related to DIC are pulmonary and central nervous system hemorrhage and thrombosis. Symptoms and signs of involvement of these systems must be carefully elicited.

Physical examination should include inspection of mucous membranes (oral, nasal), skin, venipuncture and surgical wound sites, stool, urine and any appropriate body fluids for signs of bleeding. The severity of bleeding is quantified by direct observation, calculation of transfusion requirement, fall in hematocrit, and calculation of blood-soaked dressings, or drainage, as during surgery.

Determination of bleeding at specific sites should be undertaken. If there is a question of symptoms related to the central nervous system, the cerebrospinal fluid should be examined. Careful neurologic and funduscopic exams are essential. While airway obstruction and pericardial hemorrhage are rare in DIC, these manifestations should be carefully excluded in the severely bleeding patient.

Thrombosis of blood vessels may be manifest by sudden appearance of cool limbs or accentuation in a limb of skin lesions already present. All peripheral pulses should be palpated and peripheral capillary filling evaluated. Limbs in which catheters reside are especially suspect.

Cyanosis, when occurring with DIC, should be carefully evaluated for both diagnostic and therapeutic reasons. When due to hypoxia or intense vasoconstriction secondary to hypotension, the cyanosis will clear once the underlying factors are corrected. But when the cyanosis is due to small vessel fibrin thrombi or large vessel thrombosis, complications, such as gangrene, must be anticipated. It is particularly important to examine intravascular catheter sites for evidence of thrombosis. If central venous or arterial catheters do not flush easily, have been in for substantial periods of time, or are associated with symptoms of pulmonary emboli or acral cyanosis, they should be removed. The ease of monitoring physiological information from the patient by the use of indwelling catheters must be balanced against the considerable risk of major vessel thrombosis they pose when DIC is present.

Organ and peripheral perfusion is evaluated by blood and central venous pressure, and by asking if postural hypotension, impaired mental function or reduced urinary output are present.

The laboratory evaluation of patients with DIC can be very simple. Determination of PT, platelet count, fibrinogen level and one test measuring FDP are the only necessary coagulation tests. If the diagnostic triad of prolonged PT (> 15 sec), thrombocytopenia (< 150,000/ul) and hypofibrinogenemia (< 160 mg/dl) are present, the diagnosis of DIC is established. If the triad is present but FDP are not detected (an uncommon occurrence) it is safe to assume DIC is present, while repeat tests for FDP are obtained. If only two of the screening tests are abnormal, a test of FDP must be positive to diagnose DIC. Most commonly a prolonged PT and thrombocytopenia will be associated with a normal fibrinogen level. As is shown in Chapter XII, relative hypofibrinogenemia may be present, and may be documented if previous values are much greater. When liver disease is present, additional criteria for screening tests (PT > 25 sec, platelet count < 50,000/ul, and fibrinogen level < 125 mg/dl) and tests for FDP are required to be sure of the diagnosis of DIC.

If serial coagulation test data are available the simultaneous rise in PT, fall in platelet count and fibrinogen level add further credence to the diagnosis of DIC. Other coagulation tests or tests of specific clotting factors, while useful, are not necessary for appropriate diagnosis and management of DIC.

When the diagnosis of DIC is equivocal, biopsy of a skin lesion may reveal the presence of fibrin thrombi, thus establishing the diagnosis. This test is easy to perform, but requires 2 to 24 hours for the tissue slide to be made.

Examination of the peripheral blood and bone marrow are of little aid in the diagnosis of DIC but of great help in detecting other causes of anemia and thrombocytopenia.

Other laboratory examinations of use are chest X-ray, examination of body fluids, determination of arterial pH, pCO_2, pO_2, blood culture and liver function tests. Because of the impaired hemostasis and platelet dysfunction known to occur in uremia, renal function should be evaluated.

The corner stone of the therapy is detection and correction of all precipitating and underlying diseases. Hypotension is common and must be promptly corrected. Because of bleeding and septicemia, hypovolemia should be suspected and corrected with appropriate replacement therapy. Whole blood is appropriate for hemorrhagic hypovolemia. Plasma is useful in septic states when the bleeding is minor but the hypovolemia is severe. After volume deficits have been corrected, a beta adrenergic pressor such as isoproterenol appears to be the drug of choice for treating hypotension. This was the most common pressor agent used in our series. DIC may be potentiated by alpha adrenergic agents; conversely dibenzyline, an alpha blocking agent, protects successfully in experimental DIC (213).

After other causes of impaired hemostasis are corrected, parenteral administration of vitamin K, B_{12} and folic acid is recommended, since vitamin deficiency is common in acutely ill patients. Vitamin B_{12} and folic acid are also given to correct the effect their deficiency may have on platelet production. All medications should be reviewed for possible marrow suppression or anticoagulant or antiplatelet effect and any nonessential drugs should be discontinued. Intramuscular injections in patients with DIC can be dangerous; severe hematomas frequently occur at these sites. Medications should be administered orally if possible, or alternatively in the intravenous route. In addition, venipuncture sites must be given local pressure and closely observed after a blood sample is drawn.

At present we feel heparin should be reserved for the patient with DIC who is bleeding or demonstrates thrombosis. It is also given to patients with recrudescent DIC who previously had hemorrhagic or thrombotic symptoms. Clinical trials will have to be conducted to determine if heparin is useful therapy in patients with abnormal coagulation tests but who have no clinical manifestations. If the condition precipitating DIC has already been corrected or is easily corrected (e.g. removal of a dead fetus) heparin therapy can probably be deferred. It is important to remember that correction of coagulation test abnormalities and cessation of bleeding frequently takes several days once heparin therapy has been begun. If patients are to receive large scale transfusions (hence fibrinogen and other clotting factors) heparin therapy should also be given so as to avoid the consumption of additional "fuel" by the DIC "fire". In patients who are bleeding severely, correction of coagulation factor deficits can be handled with freshly obtained whole blood or plasma, as the situation demands. In practice this is rarely needed. Factor concentrates, and fibrinogen are usually not necessary except if hepatic function is compromised. Platelet concentrates should be reserved for patients who are severely thrombocytopenic and who are bleeding into critical sites. These patients should probably always receive heparin prior to the platelet concentrates.

Once a course of therapy is begun, it is important to follow the patient for objective signs of improvement, and also for possible development of complications. We perform daily PT, platelet counts, fibrinogen levels and FDP to assess response. The level of heparin anticoagulation can be followed by the whole blood clotting time, but not by the PTT which is often prolonged due to the DIC itself. The dose is adjusted to maintain a clotting time of two to three times the normal control. Care should be taken that the blood sample for both the whole blood clotting time and the PT is obtained shortly before the next heparin dose is administered. Under these conditions circulating heparin rarely interfers with the PT determination. If the platelet count, fibrinogen level are improving but the PT is rising, over heparinization or an inadvertently heparinized blood sample should be suspected.

SPECIFIC PROBLEMS

Increased Bleeding After Initiation of Heparin Therapy

Patients with DIC commonly have increased bleeding shortly after heparin therapy is initiated (*see* Chap. XI). This is usually related to uncorrected DIC; heparin toxicity is rarely the cause. Nonetheless, any patient with increased bleeding must be carefully reevaluated. The dose of heparin administered should be checked for error. The PT, platelet count and fibrinogen levels should be determined, the status of the underlying disease and possible precipitating events considered, and possible new sites of bleeding (e.g., peptic ulcer) sought. If the coagulation tests become more abnormal or the underlying disease remains in an uncontrolled state, heparin therapy should be maintained. If the underlying disease is less severe and coagulation tests have returned towards normal, the heparin dose can be tapered or after several days discontinued. If DIC reappears, heparin can be restarted. It is important to remember in evaluating patients who bleed while receiving heparin that there is a definite time lag of two to four days before the bleeding of DIC ceases.

Management of Bleeding Following Anti-neoplastic Chemotherapy

A therapeutic dilemma arises when anti-neoplastic chemotherapy precipitates DIC and results in bleeding. DIC usually occurs one to six days after the administration of cytotoxic agents and is usually associated with massive carcinoma or leukemic cell destruction. Heparin, if added to the therapy, will usually control the bleeding while the chemotherapy is continued; coagulation tests should be performed frequently. If bleeding becomes difficult to control or is life-threatening, the need for immediate chemotherapy should be reevaluated. In addition, the possibility of superimposed septicemia or other causes of DIC must be considered.

Bleeding After Massive Transfusion

Patients with DIC often receive numerous transfusions. We usually administer one unit of blood that has been freshly drawn to every four units that are older. The fresh blood supplies platelets and labile clotting factors (particularly V and VIII) that are otherwise depleted in stored whole blood. Also, venipuncture plasma samples are checked at the bedside for evidence of gross intravascular hemolysis from an imcompatible transfusion, which in itself can precipitate DIC.

Massive Bleeding With Severe Liver Disease

The diagnosis of DIC requires additional criteria when liver disease is present (Table XIII-I). Although the liver disease itself may cause the DIC, frequently there are other precipitating factors which are amenable to treatment (e.g., septicemia). These factors should be detected and corrected. Nonvariceal bleeding is a sign that should alert the physician to the possible presence of DIC. The diagnosis and conventional management of variceal bleeding in patients with liver disease and DIC should take priority over heparin therapy with the present degree of experience.

Bleeding Associated with Abruptio Placentae and Retained Dead Fetus

These patients frequently do not require heparin therapy. Once the placenta or necrotic fetus is removed, the bleeding and DIC cease. Treatment of the underlying obstetrical problem must have the highest priority. If bleeding and/or shock persist in patients who abort, superimposed septicemia should be considered.

Bleeding With Intracranial Operations

Intracranial bleeding, particularly that associated with neurosurgical procedures, poses difficult problems in management. The mortality of DIC and CNS bleeding is high in our experience. First, the presence or absence of DIC must be established by appropriate tests. Next, signs of increased intracranial pressure must be evaluated and a decision reached concerning the need of decompressive therapy. If life-threatening signs from bleeding are present and decompression has been achieved, heparin can be administered. If the coagulation test results are markedly abnormal, fresh frozen plasma and platelet concentrates can also be given. Intracranial bleeding in patients was often associated with embolic events or concomitant invasion of blood vessels or CNS tissue by neoplastic cells or organisms.

Bleeding During Great Vessel and Cardiac Surgery

Despite the large amount of cardiovascular surgery performed at most medical centers, the occurrence of clinically significant DIC is relatively uncommon phenomenon during an operation. When bleeding does occur, it is important to recognize that it is rarely if ever due to "primary" fibrinolysis.

Differentiation of DIC from Thrombotic Thrombocytopenic Purpura (TTP)

Patient's with DIC frequently show many or all of the signs and symptoms of TTP (neurologic signs, renal failure, purpura, thrombocytopenia, schistocytosis). Often many of these signs are caused by underlying disease states that are neither related to DIC nor TTP (*see* "Organ Dysfunction", Chap. IX). Since both DIC and TTP are syndromes and not diseases and probably are caused by specific underlying diseases, it is appropriate to perform screening coagulation tests for DIC. If the tests are abnormal, the patient should be treated as though he had DIC, while a search is made to find and then treat the underlying precipitating event.

Renal Allograft Rejection

Intravascular coagulation is locally confined usually within the renal allograft that undergoes rejection. Fibrin is deposited in the kidney and FDP are excreted in the urine, but there are neither clinical manifestations of systemic bleeding, elevated serum FDP, nor other plasma coagulation changes diagnostic of DIC.

The appearance of elevated urinary FDP often signals the start of rejection. If the rejection is of the hyperacute form, classic DIC will sometimes occur, presumably due to systemic extension of the intense intrarenal clotting. Heparin should be administered. The role of heparin in the treatment of chronic rejection where changes are localized to the kidney is currently under investigation.

BIBLIOGRAPHY

1. Abildgaard, C.F.: Recognition and treatment of intravascular coagulation. *J Ped, 74:*163, 1969.
2. Abildgaard, C.F., Corrigan, J.J., Seeler, R.A., Simone, J.V., and Schulman, I.: Meningococcemia associated with intravascular coagulation. *Pediatrics, 40:*78, 1967.
3. Alkjaersig, N., Fletcher, A.P., and Sherry, S.: E-aminocaproic acid: an inhibitor of plasminogen activation. *J Biol Chem, 234:*832, 1959.
4. Bachmann, F.: Evidence for hypercoagulability in heat stroke. *J Clin Invest, 46:*1033, 1967.
5. ———: Disseminated intravascular coagulation. *Disease-a-month,* December, 1969.
6. Baker, W.B., Bang, N.U., Nachman, R.L., Raafat, F., and Horowitz, H.I.: Hypofibrinogenemic hemorrhage in acute myelogenous leukemia treated with heparin. *Ann Int Med, 61:*116, 1964.
7. Basu, H.K. and Williamson, G.F.: An unusual case of recurrent coagulation failure in pregnancy: treatment with heparin. *J Obstet Gynaecol Br Commonw, 76:*936, 1969.
8. Bayley, T., Clements, J.A., and Osbahr, A.J.: Pulmonary and circulatory effects of fibrinopeptides. *Circ Res, 21:*469, 1967.
9. Biggs, R., and Macfarland, R.G.: *Blood Coagulation and its Disorders,* 3rd ed. Philadelphia, F.A. Davis Co., 1962.
10. Birndorf, N.I., Lopas, H., and Robboy, S.J.: Disseminated intravascular coagulation and renal failure; production in the monkey with autologous red cell stroma. *Lab Invest, 25:*314, 1971.
11. Bisno, A.L., and Freeman, J.C.: The syndrome of asplenia, pneumococcal sepsis, and disseminated intravascular coagulation. *Ann Int Med, 72:*389, 1970.
12. Blix, S., and Aas, K.: Giant haemangioma, thrombocytopenia, fibrinogenpenia, and fibrinolytic activity. *Acta Med Scand, 169:*63, 1961.
13. Boyd, J.F.: Disseminated fibrin thromboembolism among stillbirths and neonatal deaths. *J Pathol Bact, 90:*53, 1965.
14. Brain, M.C.: Microangiopathic hemolytic anemia. *Ann Rev Med, 21:*133, 1970.
15. Brain, M.C., Dacie, J.V., and Hourihane, D.O'B.: Microangiopathic haemolytic anemia: the possible role of vascular lesions in pathogenesis. *Br J Haematol 8:*358, 1962.
16. Brodsky, I., and Siegel, N.H.: The diagnosis and treatment of disseminated intravascular coagulation. *Med Clin North Am, 54:*555, 1970.

17. Brodsky, I., Siegel, N.H., Kahn, S.B., Ross, E.M., and Petkov, G.: Simultaneous fibrinogen and platelet survival with (^{75}Se) selenomethionine in man: studies in diseases with normal coagulation and in hepatocellular disease with abnormal coagulation. *Br J Haematol, 18:*341, 1970.
18. Broersma, R.J., Bullemer, G.D., and Mammen, E.F.: Acidosis induced disseminated intravascular microthrombosis and its dissolution by streptokinase. *Thromb Diath Haemorrh, 24:*55, 1970.
19. Bull, B.S., and Huhn, I.N.: The production of schistocytes by fibrin strands (a scanning electron microscopic study). *Blood, 35:*104, 1970.
20. Bull, B.S., Rubenberg, M.L., Dacie, J.V., and Brain, M.C.: Microangiopathic haemolytic anaemia: mechanisms of red cell fragmentation: in vitro studies. *Br J Haematol, 14:*643, 1968.
21. Busch, G.J., Braun, W.E., Carpenter, C.B., Corson, J.M., Galvanek, E.R., Reynolds, E.S., Merrill, J.P., and Dammin, G.J.: Intravascular coagulation (IVC) in human renal allograft rejection. *Transpl Proc, 1:*267, 1969.
22. Chakrabarti, R., Bielawiec, M., Evans, J.F., and Fearnley, G.R.: Methodological study and a recommended technique for determining the euglobulin lysis time. *J Clin Pathol, 21:*698, 1968.
23. Charytan, C., and Purtilo, D.: Glomerular capillary thrombosis and acute renal failure after epsilon-amino caproic acid therapy. *N Engl J Med, 280:*1102, 1969.
24. Chernof, C.D.: Hypofibrinogenemia in scrub typhus. Report of a case. *N Engl J Med, 276:*1195, 1967.
25. Colman, R.W.: The effect of proteolytic enzymes on bovine factor V. I. Kinetics of activation and inactivation by bovine thrombin. *Biochemistry, 8:*1438, 1969.
26. ———: Activation of plasminogen by human plasma kallikrein. *Biochem Biophys Res Commun, 35:*273, 1969.
27. Colman, R.W., Braun, W.E., Busch, G.J., Dammin, G.J., and Merrill, J.P.: Coagulation studies in the hyperacute and other forms of renal-allograft rejection. *N Engl J Med, 281:*685, 1969.
28. Colman, R.W., Girey, G., Galvanek, E.G., and Busch, G.: Human renal allografts: the protective effects of heparin, kallikrein activation and fibrinolysis during hyperacute rejection. In Von Kaulla, K.N.: *Coagulation Problems in Transplanted Organs.* Springfield, Ill., Charles C Thomas, 1972, pp. 87–106.
29. Colman, R.W., Girey, G.J.D., Zacest, R., and Talamo, R.C.: The human plasma kallikrein-kinin system. In Brown, E.B., and Moore, C.V.: *Progress in Hematology.* New York, Grune & Stratton, 1971, vol. VIII, pp. 255–298.
30. Colman, R.W., and Kish, L.: Case records of the Massachusetts General Hospital (Case 29–1969). *N Engl J Med, 281:*153, 1969.
31. Colman, R.W., Mason, J.W., and Sherry, S.: The kallikreinogen-kallikrein enzyme system of human plasma. Assays of components and observations in disease states. *Ann Intern Med, 71:*763, 1969.
32. Colman, R.W., Mattler, L., and Sherry, S.: Studies on the prekallikrein (kallikreinogen)-kallikrein enzyme system of human plasma. I.

Isolation and purification of plasma kallikrein. *J Clin Invest, 48:*11, 1969.

33. ———: Studies on the prekallikrein (kallikreinogen)-kallikrein enzyme system of human plasma. II. Evidence relating the kaolin-activated arginine esterase to plasma kallikrein. *J Clin Invest, 48:*23, 1969.
34. Colman, R.W., Morris, R.E., and Osbahr, A.J.: New vasoconstrictor, bovine peptide B, released during blood coagulation. *Nature, 215:*292, 1967.
35. Colman, R.W., Oxley, L., and Giannusa, P.: Statistical comparison of the automated activated partial thromboplastin time and the clotting time in the regulation of heparin therapy. *Am J Clin Pathol, 53:*904, 1970.
36. Colman, R.W., Robboy, S.J., and Minna, J.D.: Disseminated intravascular coagulation: an approach. *Am J Med, 52:*679, 1972.
37. ———: Heparin should be used in the therapy of clinically significant disseminated intravascular coagulation. In Ingelfinger, F.J.: *Controversies in Internal Medicine.* (1974, p. 633).
38. Corrigan, J.J.Jr., and Jordan, C.M.: Heparin therapy in septicemia with disseminated intravascular coagulation. Effect on mortality and on correction of hemostatic defects. *N Engl J Med, 283:*778, 1970.
39. Corrigan, J.J.Jr., Ray, W.L., and May, N.: Changes in blood coagulation system associated with septicemia. *N Engl J Med, 279:*851, 1968.
40. Cullen, G.E., and Van Slyke, D.D.: Determination of the fibrin, globulin, and albumin nitrogen of blood plasma. *J Biol Chem, 41:*587, 1920.
41. Dennis, L.H., Eichelberger, J.W., Inman, M.M., and Conrad, M.E.: Depletion of coagulation factors in drug-resistant plasmodium falciparum malaria. *Blood, 29:*713, 1967.
42. Deykin, D.: The role of the liver in serum-induced hypercoagulability. *J Clin Invest, 45:*256, 1966.
43. ———: The clinical challenge of disseminated intravascular coagulation. *N Engl J Med, 283:*636, 1970.
44. Dieckmann, W.J.: Blood chemistry and renal function in abruptio placenta. *Am J Obstet Gynecol, 31:*734, 1936.
45. Dische, F.E., and Benfield, V.: Congenital factor VII deficiency. Haematological and genetic aspects. *Acta Haematol, 21:*257, 1959.
46. Donaldson, G.W.K., Davies, S.H., Darg, A., and Richmond, J.: Coagulation factors in chronic liver disease. *J Clin Pathol, 22:* 199, 1969.
47. Donaldson, V.H.: Mechanisms of activation of C'l esterase in hereditary angioneurotic edema plasma *in vitro.* The role of Hageman factor, a clot-promoting agent. *J Exp Med, 127:*411, 1969.
48. Doughten, R.M., and Pearson, H.A.: Disseminated intravascular coagulation associated with Aspergillus endocarditis. Fatal outcome following heparin therapy. *J Ped, 73:*576, 1968.
49. Du, J.M.H., Briggs, J.N., and Young, G.: Disseminated intravascular coagulopathy in hyaline membrane disease: massive thrombosis

following umbilical artery catheterization. *Pediatrics, 45:*287, 1970.

50. Dubber, A.H.C., McNicol, G.P., and Douglas, A.S.: Acquired hypofibrinogenaemia; "the defibrination syndrome." A study of 7 patients. *Scott Med J, 12:*138, 1967.
51. Durand, H., Aiach, M., Belaiche, J., Roge, J., Leclerc, M., and Justin-Besancon, L.: Cancer de la prostate et coagulation intravasculaire disseminee. *Sem Hop Paris, 49:*199, 1973.
52. Edson, J.R., Krivit, W., While, J.G., and Sharp, H.L.: Intravascular coagulation in acute stem cell leukemia successfully treated with heparin. *J Ped, 71:*342, 1967.
53. Ellman, L., Carvalho, A., and Colman, R.W.: The Thrombo-Wellco test as a screening test for disseminated intravascular coagulation. *N Engl J Med, 288:*633, 1973.
54. Engel, A., Alexander, B., and Pechet, L.: Activation of trypsinogen and plasminogen by thrombin preparations. *Biochemistry, 5:*1543, 1966.
55. Erdös, E.G.: Hypotensive peptides: bradykinin, kallidin and eledoisin. *Adv Pharmacol, 4:*1, 1966.
56. Evensen, S.A., Jeremic, M.: Platelets and the triggering mechanism of intravascular coagulation. *Br J Haematol, 19:*33, 1970.
57. Farbiszewski, R., Niewiarowski, S., Worowski, K., and Lipinski, B.: Release of platelet factor 4 *in vivo* during intravascular coagulation and in thrombotic states. *Thromb Diath Haemorrh, 19:*578, 1968.
58. Fleming, L.B., and Cliffton, E.E.: *In vivo* activation of the fibrinolytic system of the cat: effects of streptokinase, trypsin, and glycerol. *J Surg Res, 5:*153, 1965.
59. Fletcher, A.P., Alkjaersig, N., and Sherry, S.: Maintenance of a sustained thrombolytic state in man. I. Induction and effects. *J Clin Invest, 38:*1096, 1959.
60. ———: Pathogenesis of the coagulation defect developing during pathological plasma proteolytic ("fibrinolytic") states. I. The significance of fibrinogen proteolysis and circulating fibrinogen breakdown products. *J Clin Invest, 41:*896, 1962.
61. Fletcher, A.P., Biederman, O., Moore, D., and Alkjaersig, N.: Abnormal plasminogen-plasmin system activity (fibrinolysis) in patients with hepatic cirrhosis: its cause and consequences. *J Clin Invest, 43:*681, 1964.
62. Fox, B.: Disseminated intravascular coagulation and the Waterhouse-Friderichsen syndrome. *Arch Dis Child, 46:*680, 1971.
63. Frank, M.M., Sergent, J.S., Kane, M.A., and Alling, D.W.: Epsilon aminocaproic acid therapy of hereditary angioneurotic edema. A double blind study. *N Engl J Med, 286:*808, 1972.
64. Fulton, L.D., and Page, E.W.: Nature of the refractory state following sublethal dose of human placental thromboplastin. *Proc Soc Exp Biol Med, 68:*594, 1968.

65. Gallup, D.G., and Lucas, W.E.: Heparin treatment of consumption coagulopathy associated with intrauterine fetal death. *Obstet Gynecol, 35:*690, 1970.
66. Gans, H., and Castaneda, A.R.: Problems in hemostasis during open-heart surgery: VII. Changes in fibrinogen concentration during and after cardiopulmonary bypass with particular reference to the effect of heparin neutralization on fibrinogen. *Ann Surg, 165:*551, 1967.
67. Gaynor, E., Bouvier, C., Spaet, T.H.: Vascular lesions: possible pathogenetic basis of the generalized Shwartzman reaction. *Science, 170:*986, 1970.
68. Gigli, I., Mason, J.W., Colman, R.W., and Austen, F.K.: Interaction of kallikrein and the C'l inhibitor. *J Immunol, 104:*574, 1970.
69. Gillette, R.W., Findley, A., Conway, H.: Prolonged survival of homografts in mice treated with EACA. *Transplantation, 1:*116, 1963.
70. Girey, G.J.D., Talamo, R.C., and Colman, R.W.: The kinetics of the release of bradykinin by kallikrein by normal human plasma. *J Lab Clin Med, 77:*205, 1972.
71. Godal, H.C., and Abildgaard, C.: The symptomatic effect of anticoagulant therapy in defibrination syndrome associated with demonstrable fibrin in plasma: a case report. *Acta Med Scand, 174:*311, 1963.
72. Gollub, S., and Ulin, A.W.: Heparin-induced thrombocytopenia in man. *J Lab Clin Med, 59:*430, 1962.
73. Goodman, L.S., and Gilman, A.: *The Pharmacological Basis of Therapeutics*, 3rd ed. New York, Macmillan, 1965.
74. Gormsen, J., Fletcher, A.P., Alkjaersig, N., and Sherry, S.: Enzymic lysis of plasma clots: the influence of fibrin stabilization on lysis rates. *Arch Biochem Biophys, 120:*654, 1967.
75. Graham, J.B., Barrow, E.M., and Hougie, C.: Stuart clotting defect: II. Genetic aspects of a new hemorrhagic state. *J Clin Invest, 36:*497, 1957.
76. Gralnick, H.R., and Greipp, P.: Thrombosis with epsilon aminocaproic acid therapy. *Am J Clin Pathol, 56:*151, 1971.
77. Gralnick, H.R., and Henderson, E.: Hypofibrinogenemia and coagulation factor deficiencies with L-asparaginase treatment. *Cancer, 27:*1313, 1971.
78. Grannis, G.F.: Plasma fibrinogen: determination, normal values, physio-pathologic shifts, and fluctuations. *Clin Chem, 16:*486, 1970.
79. Haim, S., Tatarski, I., Zeltzer, M., and Amikam, E.: Disseminated intravascular coagulation presenting with cutaneous symptoms. *Dermatologica, 141:*239, 1970.
80. Hand, J.J., Kent, D.C., and Hook, V.N.: Meningococcal meningitis and meningococcemia associated with pulmonary infiltrates and hemoptysis. *Dis Chest, 54:*552, 1968.

81. Hardaway, R.M.: *Syndromes of Disseminated Intravascular Coagulation. With Special Reference to Shock and Hemorrhage.* Springfield, Charles C Thomas, 1966.
82. Hardisty, R.M., and Ingram, G.I.C.: *Bleeding Disorders: Investigation and Management.* Oxford, Blackwell Scientific Publications, 1965.
83. Hasselback, R., Marion, R.B., and Thomas, J.W.: Congenital hypofibrinogenemia in five members of a family. *Can Med Assoc J, 88:* 19, 1963.
84. Hawiger, J., Niewiarowski, S., Gurewich, V., and Thomas, D.P.: Measurement of fibrinogen and fibrin degradation products in serum by staphylococcal clumping test. *J Lab Clin Med, 75:*93, 1970.
85. Hedlin, A.M., Monkhouse, F.C.: Fibrinolytic activities of euglobulins precipitated at pH 6.4, 6.0, and 5.3. Can J Physiol Pharm, 47:935, 1969.
86. Ingram, G.I.C., and Matchett, M.O.: A rapid "side-room" method for the determination of plasma fibrinogen concentration as fibrin. *J Clin Pathol, 13:*469, 1960.
87. Johnson, A.J., and Merskey, C.: Diagnosis of diffuse intravascular clotting: its relation to secondary fibrinolysis and treatment with heparin. *Thromb Diath Haemorrh Suppl, 20:*161, 1966.
88. Kaplan, A.P., and Austin, K.F.: A prealbumin activator of prekallikrein. II. Derivation of activators of prekallikrein from active Hageman factor by digestion with plasmin. *J Exp Med, 133:*696, 1971.
89. Katz, J., Lurie, A., Becker, D., and Metz, J.: The euglobulin lysis time test: an ineffectual monitor of the therapeutic inhibition of fibrinolysis. *J Clin Path, 23:*529, 1970.
90. Kazemi, H., and Kline, I.K.: Case records of the Massachusetts General Hospital (Case 38–1969). *N Engl J Med, 281:*666, 1969.
91. Kellermeyer, R.W., and Graham, R.C. Jr.: Kinins—possible physiologic and pathologic roles in man. *N Engl J Med, 279:*754, 1968.
92. Kincaid-Smith, P., Laver, M.C., and Fairley, K.F.: Dipyridamole and anticoagulants in renal disease due to glomerular and vascular lesions: a new approach to therapy. *Med J Aust, 1:*145, 1970.
93. Klein, R., and Robboy, S.J.: Case records of the Massachusetts General Hospital (Case 7–1973). *N Engl J Med, 288:*363, 1973.
94. Konttinen, Y.P.: *Fibrinolysis: Chemistry, Physiology, Pathology and Clinics.* Tampere, Finland: Oy Star Ab, 1968.
95. Korsan-Bengtsen, K., Ysander, L., Blohme, G., and Tibblin, E.: Extensive muscle necrosis after long-term treatment with aminocaproic acid (EACA) in a case of hereditary periodic edema. *Acta Med Scand, 185:*341, 1969.
96. Kowalski, E.: Fibrinogen derivatives and their biologic activities. *Sem Hematol 5:*45, 1968.

97. Kowalski, E., Kopec, M., and Niewiarowski, S.: An evaluation of the euglobulin method for the demonstration of fibrinolysis. *J Clin Path, 12:*215, 1959.
98. Krevans, J.R., Jackson, D.P., Conley, C.L., and Hartman, R.C.: The nature of the hemorrhagic disorder accompanying hemolytic transfusion reactions in man. *Blood, 12:*834, 1957.
99. Kwaan, H.C., and Astrup, T.: Tissue repair in the presence of locally applied inhibition of fibrinolysis. *Exp Mol Pathol. 11:*82, 1969.
100. Lasch, H.G., Heene, D.L., Huth, K., and Sandritter, W.: Pathophysiology, clinical manifestations and therapy of consumption-coagulopathy ("Verbrauchs-koagulopathie"). *Am J Cardiol, 20:*381, 1967.
101. Lasch, H.G., Krecke, H.J., Rodriquez-Erdman, F., Sesser, H.H., and Schulterle, G.: Verbrauchs koagulopathie (Pathogenese und therapie). *Folia Haematol N F, 61:*325, 1961.
102. Leavey, R.A., Kahn, S.B., and Brodsky, I.: Disseminated intravascular coagulation, a complication of chemotherapy in acute myelomonocytic leukemia. *Cancer, 26:*142, 1970.
103. Loeliger, E.A., Van, D.E., Esch, B., Cleton, F.J., Booij, H.L., and Mattern: On the metabolism of factor VII. *Proc 7th Cong Int Soc Hematol, London, 2:*764, 1959.
104. Lever, W.F.: *Histopathology of the Skin,* 4th ed. Philadelphia, Lippincott, 1967.
105. Liban, E., and Raz, S.: A clinicopathologic study of fourteen cases of amniotic fluid embolism. *Am J Clin Path, 51:*477, 1966.
106. Little, J.R.: Purpura fulminans treated successfully with anticoagulation. *JAMA, 169:*104, 1959.
107. Lopas, H., Birndorf, N.I., Bell, C.E., Robboy, S.J., Fortwengler, H.P., and Biddison, H.P.: Experimental transfusion reactions in monkeys: hemolytic and renal effects of isoimmune transfused IgG and IgM. *Br J Haematol, 23:*765, 1972.
108. Lopas, H., Birndorf, N.I., Bell, C.E., Robboy, S.J., and Colman, R.W.: Immune hemolytic transfusion reactions in monkeys: activation of the kallikrein system. *Am J Physiol, 225:*372(1973).
109. Lopas, H., Birndorf, N.I., Robboy, S.J.: Experimental transfusion reactions and disseminated intravascular coagulation produced by incompatible plasma in monkeys. *Transfusion, 11:*196, 1971.
110. Lowney, E.D.: Effects of epsilon-aminocaproic acid on the tuberculin reaction in man. *J Invest Dermatol, 42:*243, 1964.
111. McCreary, T., and Wurzel, H.: Poisonous snake bites. Report of a case. *JAMA, 170:*268, 1959.
112. McGehee, W.B., Rapaport, S.I., and Hjort, P.F.: Intravascular coagulation in fulminant meningococcemia. *Ann Int Med, 67:*250, 1967.
113. McGovern, V.J.: The pathophysiology of gram-negative septicaemia. *Pathology, 4:*265, 1972.
114. McGrath, J.M., and Stewart, G.J.: The effects of endotoxin on vascular endothelium. *J Exp Med, 129:*833, 1969.

115. McKay, D.G.: *Disseminated Intravascular Coagulation.* New York, Harper & Row, 1965.
116. ———: Progress in disseminated intravascular coagulation. *Calif Med, 111:*186, 279, 1970.
117. ———: Participation of components of the blood coagulation system in the inflammatory response. *Am J Path, 67:*181, 1972.
118. McKay, D.G., and Margaretten, W.: Disseminated intravascular coagulation in virus diseases. *Arch Intern Med, 120:*129, 1967.
119. McKay, D.G., and Müller-Berghaus, G.: Therapeutic implications of disseminated intravascular coagulation. *Am J Cardiol, 20:*392, 1967.
120. McNicol, G.P., Fletcher, A.P., Alkjaersig, N., and Sherry, S.: The use of epsilon aminocaproic acid, a potent inhibitor of fibrinolytic activity in the management of postoperative hematuria. *J Urol, 86:*829, 1961.
121. ———: The absorption, distribution and excretion of e-aminocaproic acid following oral or intravenous administration to man. *J Lab Clin Med, 59:*15, 1962.
122. Mainwaring, D., and Keidan, S.E.: Fibrinolysis in haemophilia. The effect of epsilon aminocaproic acid. *Br J Haemat, 11:*682, 1965.
123. Marcus, A.J.: The role of lipids in blood coagulation. *Adv Lipid Res, 4:*1, 1966.
124. Marder, V.J., Matchett, M.O., and Sherry, S.: Detection of serum fibrinogen and fibrin degradation products. *Am J Med, 51:*71, 1971.
125. Marder, V.J., and Shulman, N.R.: High molecular weight derivatives of human fibrinogen produced by plasmin. II. Mechanism of their anticoagulant activity. *J Biol Chem, 244:*2120, 1969.
126. Marder, V.J., Shulman, N.R., and Carroll, W.R.: High molecular weight derivatives of human fibrinogen produced by plasmin. I. Physicochemical and immunological characterization. *J Biol Chem, 244:*2111, 1969.
127. Mason, J.W., and Colman, R.W.: The role of Hageman factor in disseminated intravascular coagulation induced by septicemia, neoplasia, or liver disease. *Thromb Diath Haemorrh, 26:*325, 1971.
128. Mason, J.W., Kleeberg, U., Dolan, P., and Colman, R.W.: Plasma kallikrein and Hageman factor in gram negative bacteremia. *Ann Intern Med, 73:*545, 1970.
129. Merrills, R.J., and Shaw, J.T.B.: Kinetics of fibrin clot lysis. *Biochem J, 106:*101, 1968.
130. Merskey, C., Johnson, A.J., Kleiner, G.J., and Wohl, H.: The defibrination syndrome: clinical features and laboratory diagnosis. *Br J Haematol, 13:*528, 1967.
131. Merskey, C., Kleiner, G.J., and Johnson, A.J.: Quantitative estimation of split products of fibrinogen in human serum, relation to diagnosis and treatment. *Blood, 28:*1, 1966.

132. Miller, S.P.: Coagulation dynamics in Factor V deficiency: a family study with a note on the occurrence of thrombophlebitis. *Thromb Diath Haemorrh, 13:*500, 1965.
133. Mills, J.A.: Systemic vasculitis. In Fitzpatrick, T.B., Arndt, K.A., Clark, J.H. Jr., Eisen, A.Z., Van Scott, E.J., and Vaughan, J.H.: Dermatology and General Medicine. New York, McGraw Hill, pp. 1481–1493, 1971.
134. Mokarhan, S., Gajewski, J., Grace, N., Greenberg, M., Iber, F., and Gurewich, V.: Association of consumption coagulopathy with bleeding in cirrhosis. *Clin Res, 19:*399, 1971.
135. Mosesson, M.W., Colman, R.W., and Sherry, S.: Chronic intravascular coagulation syndrome. Report of a case with special studies of an associated plasma cryoprecipitate ("Cryofibrinogen"). *N Engl J Med, 278:*815, 1968.
136. Müller-Berghaus, G., and McKay, D.G.: Prevention of the generalized Shwartzman reaction in pregnant rats by α-adrenergic blocking agents. *Lab Invest, 17:*276, 1967.
137. Mustard, J.F., and Packham, M.A.: Thromboembolism: a manifestation of the response of blood to injury. *Circulation, 42:*1, 1970.
138. Myers, A.R., Colman, R.W., and Bloch, K.J.: Fibrinogen degradation products in sera of patients with systemic lupus erythematosus. *Arthritis Rheum, 12:*318, 1969.
139. Myhre-Jensen, O., Hansen, E.S., and Buttrago, B.: Renal microthrombosis. Incidence in 500 consecutive autopsies, clinicopathological relations. *Acta Pathol Microbiol Scand* [A], *80:*403, 1972.
140. Nachnani, G.H., Lessin, L.S., Motomiya, T., and Jensen, W.N.: Scanning electron microscopy of thrombogenesis on vascular catheter surfaces. *N Engl J Med, 286:*139, 1972.
141. Naeye, R.L.: Thrombotic state after hemorrhagic diathesis; possible complication of therapy with epsilon aminocaproic acid. *Blood, 19:*694, 1962.
142. Najjar, S.S., and Ahmad, M.: Heparin therapy in fulminant meningococcemia. *J Ped, 75:*449, 1969.
143. Nasagawa, S., Takahashi, H., Koida, M., and Suzuki, T.: Partial purification of bovine plasma kallikreinogen, its activation by the Hageman factor. *Biochem Biophys Res Commun, 32:*644, 1968.
144. Natelson, E.A., Lynch, E.C., Alfrey, C.P.Jr., and Gross, J.B.: Heparin induced thrombocytopenia; an unexpected response to treatment of comsumption coagulopathy. *Ann Intern Med, 71:*1121, 1969.
146. Niemetz, J., and Nossel, H.L.: Activated coagulation factors: *in vivo* and *in vitro* studies. *Br J Haematol, 16:*337, 1969.
147. Nies, A.S., Forsyth, R.P., Williams, H.E., and Melmon, K.L.: Contribution of kinins to endotoxin shock in unanesthetized Rhesus monkeys, *Circ Res, 22:*155, 1968.
148. Niewiarowski, S.: Detection of fibrinogen derivatives in plasma and

in serum and its significance in the diagnosis of intravascular coagulation and fibrinolysis. In *French Congress of Anaestheology, (Symposium on Fibrinolysis and Defibrination)*, Librairie Arnette, Paris, pp. 67–84, 1973.

149. Niewiarowski, S., Nandi, M., Colman, R.W., and Bloch, K.: Electrophoretic pattern and reactivity of fibrinogen degradation products (FDP) in three assays. *Scand J Haematol, 8* (supp 13): 129, 1970.
150. Niewiarowski, S., and Prou-Wartelle, O.: Role du facteur contact (facteur Hageman) dans la fibrinolyse. *Thromb Diath Haemorrh, 3:*593, 1954.
151. Nilsson, I.M., Andersson, L., and Bjorkman, S.E.: Epsilon aminocaproic acid (EACA) as a therapeutic agent based on 5 years clinical experience. *Acta Med Scand, 180* (supp 448):1, 1966.
152. Nossel, H.L., Niemetz, J., Waxman, S.A., and Spector, S.L.: Defibrination syndrome in a patient with chronic thrombocytopenic purpura. *Am J Med, 46:*591, 1969.
153. Ogston, D., Bennett, N.B., Ogston, C.M.: The fibrinolytic enzyme system in hepatic cirrhosis and malignant metastases. *J Clin Path, 24:*822, 1971.
154. Ogston, D., Ogston, C.M., Ratnoff, O.D., and Forbes, C.D.: Studies on a complex mechanism for the activation of plasminogen by kaolin and by chloroform: the participation of Hageman factor and additional cofactors. *J Clin Invest, 48:*1786, 1959.
155. O'Meara, R.A.Q.: Coagulative properties of cancers. *Ir J Med Sci, 6:*474, 1958.
156. Oski, F.A., and Naiman, J.L.: Effect of live measles vaccine on the platelet count. *N Engl J Med, 275:*352, 1966.
157. Pederson, H.J., Tebo, T.H., and Johnson, S.A.: Evidence of hemolysis in the initiation of hemostasis. *Am J Clin Path, 48:*62, 1967.
158. Peterson, E.P., and Taylor, H.B.: Amniotic fluid embolism, an analysis of 40 cases. *Obstet Gynecol, 35:*787, 1970.
159. Philippidis, P., Naiman, J.L., Sibinga, M.S., and Valdes-Dapnea, M.A.: Disseminated intravascular coagulation in Candida albicans septicemia. *J Ped, 78:*683, 1971.
160. Pitney, W.R., Pettit, J.E., and Armstrong, L.: Control of heparin therapy. *Br Med J, 4:*139, 1970.
161. Pittman, G.R., Senhauser, D.A., and Lowney, J.F.: Acute promyelocytic leukemia. A report of 3 autopsied cases. *Am J Clin Path, 46:*214, 1966.
162. Point, W., and Castleman, B.: Case records of the Massachusetts General Hospital (Case 24–1970). *N Engl J Med, 282:*1310, 1970.
163. Polliack, A.: Acute promyelocytic leukemia with disseminated intravascular coagulation. *Am J Clin Pathol, 56:*155, 1971.
164. Preston, F.E., Malia, R.G., Sworn, M.J., and Blackburn, E.K.: Intravascular coagulation and E. coli septicaemia. *J Clin Pathol, 26:*120, 1973.

165. Quick, A.J.: *Hemorrhagic Diseases and Thrombosis*, 2nd ed. Philadelphia, Lea and Febiger, 1966.
166. Rake, M.O., Flute, P.T., Pannell, G., and Williams, R.: Intravascular coagulation in acute hepatic necrosis. *Lancet, 1:*533, 1970.
167. Rand, J.J., Moloney, W.C., and Sise, H.S.: Coagulation defects in acute promyelocytic leukemia. *Arch Int Med, 123:*39, 1969.
168. Ratnoff, O.D.: Epsilon aminocaproic acid—a dangerous weapon. *N Engl J Med, 280:*1124, 1969.
169. Ratnoff, O.D., and Menzie, C.: A new method for the determination of fibrinogen in small samples of plasma. *J Lab Clin Med, 37:*316, 1951.
170. Robbins, J., and Stetson, C.A.: An effect of antigen-antibody interaction on blood coagulation. *J Exp Med, 109:*1, 1959.
171. Robboy, S.J., Colman, R.W., and Minna, J.D.: Fibrinolysis versus disseminated intravascular coagulation. *N Engl J Med, 281:*222, 1969.
172. ———: Pathology of disseminated intravascular coagulation (DIC): analysis of twenty-six cases. *Hum Pathol, 3:*327, 1972.
173. Robboy, S.J., Mihm, M.C., Colman, R.W., and Minna, J.D.: The skin in disseminated intravascular coagulation (DIC): prospective analysis of 36 cases. *Br J Derm, 88:*221, 1973.
174. Robboy, S.J., Minna, J.D., Colman, R.W.: Resolution of pathological fibrinolysis with heparin. *Clin Res, 18:*414, 1970.
175. Robboy, S.J., Minna, J.D., Colman, R.W., Birndorf, N.I., and Lopas, H.: Pulmonary hemorrhage syndrome as a manifestation of disseminated intravascular coagulation: analysis of 10 cases. *Chest, 63:*718, 1973.
176. Robboy, S.J., Salisbury, K., Ragsdale, B., Bobroff, L.M., Jacobson, B.M., and Colman, R.W.: Mechanism of aspergillus-induced microangiopathic hemolytic anemia. *Arch Intern Med, 128:*790, 1971.
177. Rodriguez-Erdman, F.: Bleeding due to increased intravascular blood coagulation: hemorrhagic syndromes caused by consumption of blood-clotting factors (consumption-coagulopathies). *N Engl J Med, 273:*1370, 1965.
178. Roos, J., Van Arkel, C., Verloop, M.C., and Jordan, F.L.J.: A "new" family with Stuart-Prower deficiency. *Thromb Diath Haemorrh, 3:*59, 1959.
179. Rosenthal, R.L.: Acute promyelocytic leukemia associated with hypofibrinogenemia. *Blood, 21:*495, 1963.
180. Saldeen, T.: The importance of intravascular coagulation and inhibition of the fibrinolytic system in experimental fat embolism. *J Trauma, 10:*287, 1970.
181. Schapiro, R.H., Castleman, B., and Robboy, S.J.: Case records of the Massachusetts General Hospital (Case 44–1970). *N Engl J Med, 283:*919, 1970.
182. Schneider, C.L.: "Fibrin embolism" (disseminated intravascular

coagulation) with defibrination as one of the end results of placenta abruption. *Surg Gynecol Obstet, 92:*27, 1951.

183. Semar, M., Skoza, L., Johnson, A.J.: Partial purification and properties of a plasminogen activator from human erythrocytes. *J Clin Invest, 48:*1777, 1969.
184. Shanberge, J.N., Tanaka, K., Gruhl, M.C.: Chronic consumption coagulopathy due to hemangiomatous transformation of the spleen. *Am J Clin Path, 56:*723, 1971.
185. Sherry, S.: Fibrinolysis. *Am Rev Med, 19:*247, 1968.
186. Simone, J.V.: Disseminated intravascular coagulation. *Adv Intern Med, 15:*339, 1969.
187. Sohal, R.S., Sun, S.C., Colcolough, H.L., and Burch, G.E.: Heat stroke. An electron microscopic study of endothelial cell damage and disseminated intravascular coagulation. *Arch Intern Med, 122:* 43, 1968.
188. Spaet, T.H.: Hemostatic homeostasis. *Blood, 28:*112, 1966.
189. Spittell, J.A. Jr.: Reynaud's phenomenon and allied vasopastic conditions, and diseases of the vascular system related to environmental temperature. In Fairbairn, J.F. III, Juergens, J.L., and Spittel, J.A. Jr.: *Peripheral Vascular Disease.* Philadelphia, Saunders, 1972, pp. 387–420, 421–439.
190. Starzl, T.E., Boehmig, H.J., Amemiya, H., Wilson, C.B., Dixon, F.J., Giles, G.R., Simpson, K.M., and Halgrimson, C.G.: Clotting changes, including disseminated intravascular coagulation, during rapid renal-homograft rejection. *N Engl J Med, 283:*383, 1970.
191. Steiger, B., White, J.G., and Krivit, W.: Epsilon aminocaproic acid for hematuria in hemophilia. *Lancet, 82:*421, 1962.
192. Stiehm, E.R., and Damrosch, D.S.: Factors in the prognosis of meningococcal infection. *J Ped, 68:*457, 1966.
193. Stossel, T.P., and Levy, R.: Intravascular coagulation associated with pneumoccal bacteremia and symmetrical peripheral gangrene. *Arch Intern Med, 125:*876, 1970.
194. Straub, P.W., Riedler, G., and Frick, P.G.: Hypofibrinogenaemia in metastatic carcinoma of the prostate: suppression of systemic fibrinolysis by heparin. *J Clin Path, 20:*152, 1967.
195. Strauss, H.S., Kevy, S.V., and Diamond, L.K.: Ineffectiveness of prophylactic epsilon aminocaproic acid in severe hemophilia. *N Engl J Med, 273:*301, 1965.
196. Swartz, J.H., Medrek, T.F., and Robboy, S.J.: A new stain for systemic fungi in tissue. *Am J Clin Path, 57:*27, 1972.
197. Taylor, F.B. Jr., and Funderberg, H.: Inhibition of the C'l component of complement by amino acids. *Immunology, 7:*319, 1964.
198. Thomas, D.P., Niewiarowski, S., Myers, A.R., Block, K.J., and Colman, R.W.: A comparative study of four methods for detecting fibrinogen degradation products from patients with various diseases. *N Engl J Med, 283:*663, 1970.

199. Thomas, D.P., Ream, V.J., and Stuart, R.K.: Platelet aggregation in patients with Laennec's cirrhosis of the liver. *N Engl J Med, 276:*1344, 1967.
200. Thomas, J.W., Hasselback, R.C., and Perry, W.H.: A study of the haemorrhagic diathesis in leukaemia and allied diseases. *Can Med Assoc J, 83:*639, 1960.
201. Thomas, L., Denney, F.W., and Floyd, J.: Studies on the generalized Shwartzman reaction. III. Lesions of the myocardium and coronary artery accompanying the reaction in rabbits prepared by infection with group A staphylococci. *J Exp Med, 92:*751, 1953.
202. Triantaphyllopoulos, D.C.: Intravascular coagulation following injection of prothrombin complex. *Am J Clin Path, 57:*603, 1972.
203. Tytgat, G.N.: Accelerated fibrinogen consumption in cirrhosis of the liver. *Clin Res, 18:*419, 1970.
204. Tytgat, G.N., Collen, D., and Verstraete, M.: Metabolism of fibrinogen in cirrhosis of the liver. *J Clin Invest, 50:*1690, 1971.
205. Umlas, J.: Glomeruloid structures in thrombohemolytic thrombocytopenic purpura, glomerulonephritis, and disseminated intravascular coagulation. *Hum Pathol, 3:*437, 1972.
206. Umlas, J., and Kaiser, J.: Thrombohemolytic thrombocytopenic purpura (TTP): a disease or a syndrome? *Am J Med, 49:*723, 1970.
207. Verstraete, M., Amery, A., Vermylen, C., and Robyn, G.: Heparin treatment of bleeding. *Lancet, 1:*446, 1963.
208. Verstraete, M., Vermylen, C., Vermylen, J., and Vandenbroucke, J.: Excessive consumption of blood coagulation components as cause of hemorrhagic diathesis. *Am J Med, 38:*899, 1965.
209. Walsh, R.T., and Barnhart, M.I.: Clearance of coagulation and fibrinolysis products by the reticuloendothelial system. *Thromb Diath Haemorrh, 22* (supp 36):83, 1969.
210. Webber, A.J., and Johnson, S.A.: Platelet participation in blood coagulation; aspects of hemostasis. *Am J Pathol, 60:*19, 1970.
211. Wessler, S.: Studies in intravascular coagulation. III. The pathogenesis of serum-induced venous thrombosis. *J Clin Invest, 34:*647, 1955.
212. Wessler, S., and Yin, E.T.: On the mechanism of thrombosis. In Brown, E.B., and Moore, C.V.: *Progress in Hematology.* New York, Grune & Stratton, 1969, vol. VI, pp. 201–232.
213. Whitaker, A.N., McKay, D.G., and Csavossy, I.: Studies of catecholamine shock. I. Disseminated intravascular coagulation. *Am J Pathol, 56:*153, 1969.
214. Wigger, H.J., Bransilver, B.R., and Blanc, W.A.: Thromboses due to catheterization in infants and children. *J Ped, 76:*1, 1970.
215. Wilner, G.D., Nossel, H.L., and LeRoy, E.C.: Activation of Hageman factor by collagen. *J Clin Invest, 47:*2608, 1968.
216. Winkelstein, A., Songster, C.L., Caras, T.S., Berman, H.H., and West, W.L.: Fulminant meningococcemia and disseminated intravascular coagulation. *Arch Int Med, 124:*55, 1969.

217. Wycoff, H.D.: Production of fibrinogen following an endotoxin injection. *Proc Soc Exp Biol Med, 133:*940, 1970.
218. Yamagata, S., Mori, K., Kayaba, T., Hiratsuka, I., Kitamura, T., Ishimori, A., Takahashi, O., Tozawa, Y., Matsuyama, K., and Toyohara, M.: A case of congenital afibrinogenemia and review of reported cases in Japan. *Tohoku J Exp Med, 96:*15, 1968.
219. Yin, E.T., Wessler, S., and Stoll, P.J.: Rabbit plasma inhibitor of the activated species of blood coagulation factor X. Purification and some properties. *J Biol Chem, 246:*3694, 1971.
220. ———: Biological properties of the naturally occurring plasma inhibitor to activated factor X. *J Biol Chem, 246:*3703, 1971.
221. Yoshikawa, T., Tanaka, K.R., and Guze, L.B.: Infection and disseminated intravascular coagulation. *Medicine, 50:*237, 1971.
222. Zachariae, H., Malmquist, J., Oates, J.A., and Pettinger, W.: Studies on the mechanism of kinin formation in inflammation. *J Physiol, 190:*81, 1967.

PATIENT INDEX

AUTHOR INDEX

SUBJECT INDEX

C